gourmet food with all of the flavor and none of the guilt

THE GUILT FREE GOURMET

Low Fat & Calorie Cookbook - Volume 3
GOURMET BURGERS, SANDWICHES & SIDES

D1736551

Follow me online at:

The Web: www.theguiltfreegourmet.net
Connect: *@dhallakx7*
Facebook: The Guilt Free Gourmet LLC.
Instagram: TheGuiltFreeGourmet ... No, seriously... Follow me on Instagram!!
Youtube Channel: The Guilt Free Gourmet

LEGAL DISCLAIMERS:

The Guilt Free Gourmet® 2020

Though we have copyright protection over this publication and the materials here-in,
we at The Guilt Free Gourmet want to make sure you understand that **you have
our full and complete permission to have this material printed for your private use**!
**If you are a home cook or a cooking enthusiast, please know that we wish for you to be able
to print this material, either at home, or at a business that offers printing services, such as
Staples, Office Depot, Kinkos, etc.**

If you try to take this to a printing center and they say that they can't print it,
PLEASE tell them to look at the disclaimer cited above. The Author has expressly
stated that he (me) has given permission for you to print it... Then poke him/her in the
chest to establish dominance. Howling loudly while pointing at their copy machine.

Weight Watchers International & WW ®

The Guilt Free Gourmet is not affiliated with, nor is it endorsed by
Weight Watchers International, Inc. (now WW®). Weight Watchers has not reviewed
this publication for accuracy or suitability for WW members.

Weight Watchers, WW®, Point, Points, Smart Points, SP's and Freestyle are all registered
trademarks of Weight Watchers International, Inc. Authentic information about
the program is only available at your local WW workshop or online through the
WW website and mobile app. The information and recipes contained within this guide
are based solely on the recollections and assumptions of The Guilt Free Gourmet.
The information and recipes are not warranted for any purpose by the author other
than for educational purposes and for reference under fair use doctrine.

All readers are encouraged to go to a WW Workshop or the WW website for actual WW information
and to also enter the listed ingredients of my recipes themselves into the Recipe Builder. Point
values for certain ingredients change and are updated periodically by WW®, which may
change the point values we are suggesting to be accurate for our recipes at this time.

This guide is in **NO WAY** meant to be a replacement for the WW Program. It is merely
developed and intended for use as a collection of privately developed recipes,
designed to complement the instructional materials and resources
provided by WW to its members... BECAUSE WW IS AWESOME!

Any non-generic recipes within this guide were developed by me.
All Point values were determined by entering the ingredients, measurements and
servings into the Recipe Builder within the WW mobile App that is only
available to paying members of the system. I strongly encourage anyone interested
in developing a healthier lifestyle to join and follow the strategies for healthy living
provided by Weight Watchers International (WW®).

All use of the terms Weight Watchers, WW, Point, Points, Smart Points, SP's and Freestyle
in the following cookbook are used SOLELY for reference purposes,
as is appropriate and allowed under fair use doctrine.

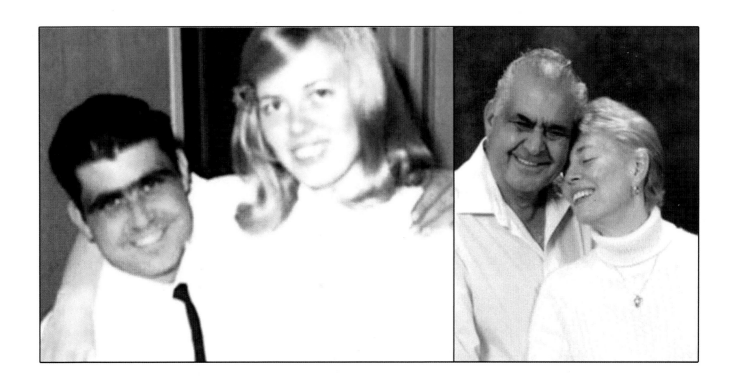

Dedicated to my Mom & Dad.
King Louie & The Yellow Rose of Texas
I miss'ya Mom.

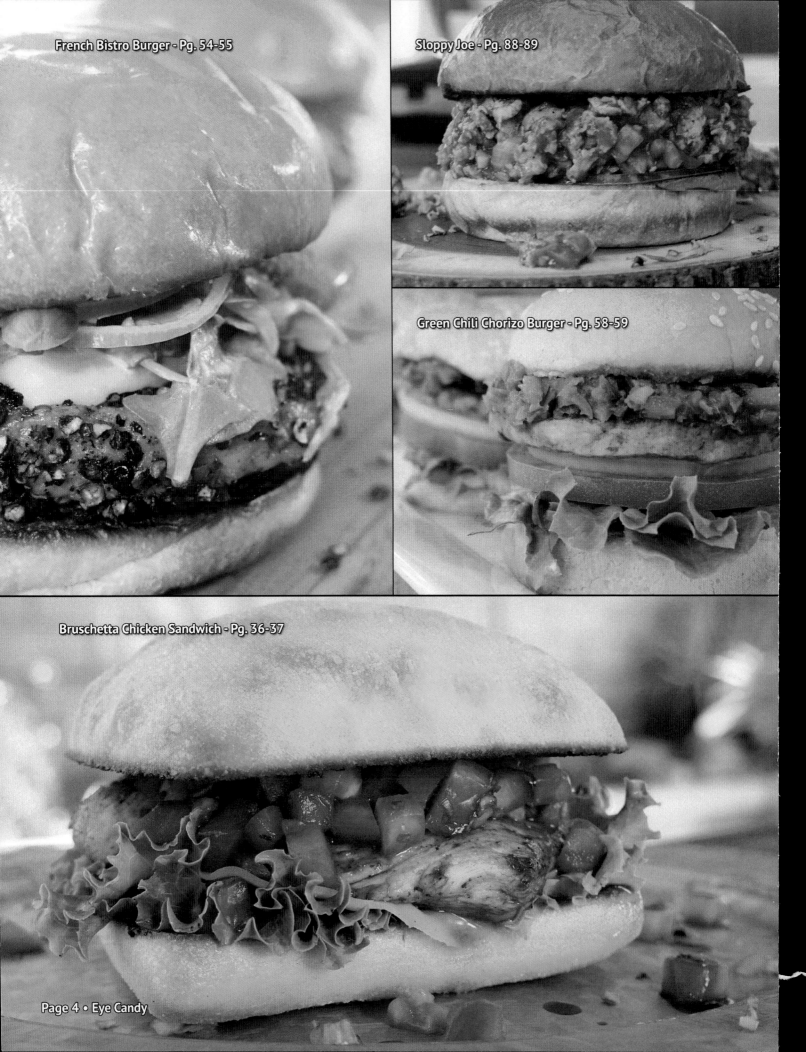

French Bistro Burger - Pg. 54-55

Sloppy Joe - Pg. 88-89

Green Chili Chorizo Burger - Pg. 58-59

Bruschetta Chicken Sandwich - Pg. 36-37

Table of Contents

2020 | Cookbook Volume 3 - 1st Edition
Low Fat & Calorie Gourmet Burgers, Sandwiches & Sides

Introduction

My personal weight loss journey and why
I started trying to cook healthier ... *pages 6-7*

Recipe Reminder

There are recipes that are referenced in this book, that are actually located in my 2 prior Cookbooks. This page explains how you can easily access them for free online, or how to get a printed copy ... *page 8*

Important Kitchen Gadgets

Highlighting some of the kitchen gadgets I used to make these recipes. They aren't required, but they do make things a bit easier ... *page 9*

Important Ingredients

Pointing out a few of the key ingredients used in these recipes, as well as important considerations ... *pages 10 - 11*

Condiments, Dressings & Spreads

Recipes for 29 of the low calorie & low 'Point' dressings, sauces and spreads used in this book's dishes. Also included is a page explaining ingredient substitutions for the different condiments ... *pages 12 - 21*

Burgers & Sandwiches

36 delicious and **GOURMET**, low calorie, low fat, low 'Point' burgers and sandwiches. These are not 'diet food' burgers. These are insane burgers and sandwiches that you would be excited to order at a restaurant. They are big, hearty portions that are filling, satisfying... and miraculously, they also promote healthy weight loss ... *pages 22 - 97*

Baked Parmesan Carrot Fries - pg. 106

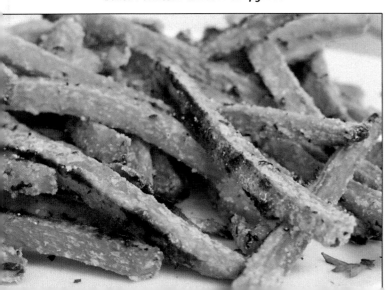

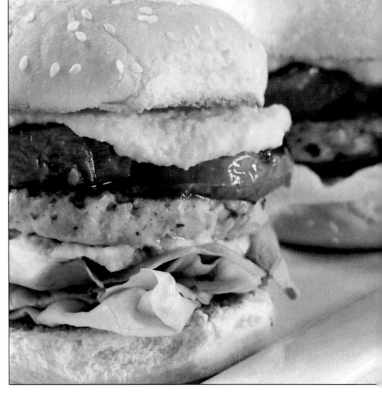

Lebanese Kafta Burger with Roasted Tomatoes - pg. 66 - 67

Side Dishes & Salads

19 low calorie, low fat and low-ish 'Point' side dishes and salads. Everything from Loaded Mac n Cheese, Onion Rings and Baked Beans, to Mexican 'Street Corn' and Potato Salad ... *pages 98 - 113*

Bonus Recipes

Because this book has a 'backyard burger party' vibe to it, I wanted to include a couple of extra recipes. From how to make low calorie & 'Point' burger buns, to easy peach cobbler, cucumber mint lemonade, peanut butter & jelly cake and more ... *pages 114 - 121*

Happy Little Burgers & Acknowledgements

Before I make a swift exit, like the 'Hamburglar', I should probably thank a few folks for their encouragement during this whole process ... *pages 122 - 123*

Nutritional Information

A 2 page spread, with the nutritional values for every recipe in the book. Information provided by the borderline insane, *@cake.riot* ... *pages 124 - 125*

Book Index

Need help finding recipes in a flash? This organized list of all the recipes will help you hitch a ride on my culinary crazy train ... *pages 126 - 127*

Introduction

Alright, for you folks that already have my other 2 cookbooks, or follow me on Connect, this is going to be preeeeetty repetitive. Sorry *shrugs* This introduction is mainly for the folks that don't know me yet.

Hi there, my name is Daniel, but most of you know me from **WW Connect** as '**Dhallakx7**'. As of the writing of this cookbook, I'm a 43-year-old stay at home dad to my 2 special needs kidlettes, Rachel (Autistic) and Jesse (Down Syndrome). Prior to this, I worked as a Graphic Designer & Web Developer for a really great company. I had just received a promotion, but when Jesse was born preemie and his diagnosis was finally confirmed, our priorities had to change, so I became Mr. Mom.

I still remember the night in 3rd grade when I turned from liking food, to wanting to gorge on food. My best friend Bart and I went to a high school soccer game with my older brother. At that game I saw something that I'd never seen before. A food vendor showed up in the bleachers pushing a food cart. He was using it to make hot, sugar coated mini cake donuts, fresh to order. I remember running down to that cart with my friend, looking at the fresh donuts, then immediately running up to my brother and asking for the money to buy some... then to buy some more... then to buy some more. And that's where it started.

I spent the better part of the next 30 years going from "husky" to overweight, eventually becoming heavy enough to be classified as obese. I only went swimming 3 or 4 times in the past 25 years out of shame for how I looked. I would make excuses not to see friends who were visiting from out of town, whom I hadn't seen in years. Heck, I wouldn't even change in the same room as my wife because I was

The new and improved 2020 Dad Bod GTO. Now available with dual child carriers, improved mileage and extended warranty

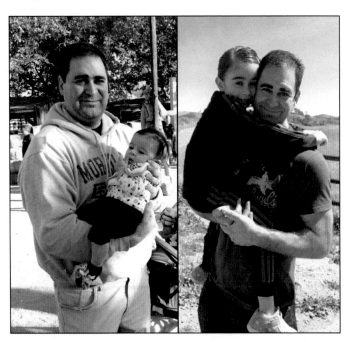

embarrassed about my body. Yet, did it make me want to change and lose weight? Nope, I figured it wasn't worth it.

In order to lose weight, I was going to be eating nothing but rice cakes and tasteless diet food. I would have to start going to the gym, running and stop eating all the foods that I loved to eat. People on diets are always so miserable and complain about what they can't eat, how their diet de jour doesn't allow them to have sugar, or they are cutting all carbs, or they are doing "cleanses" or whatever insane dietary deprivation is the current trend. Why in the heck would I want to do that? I'd rather be fat and eating than be skinny and surviving on rice cakes, bean curd and sadness. But, when I finally hit my mental rock bottom, I stumbled upon an article online late at night. It was written by a female blogger who tried Weight Watchers for one month without doing any exercise and without giving up eating regular food. She ended up losing 5 pounds over the course of the month without working out, while still eating normal foods and staying within her Weight Watchers daily allotment of "Smart Points". I figured it was worth a shot as I had no

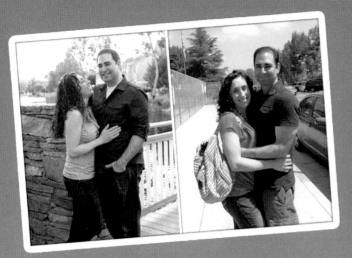

Don't let food manipulate you, learn to manipulate your food

Rethink How You Cook

- Lower the fat, calories, sugar and carbs of foods, by swapping out high fat & calorie ingredients.
- Lose weight, by turning high fat & calorie food that you love, into a leaner and healthier dish.
- Retrain your brain to automatically think of ingredient substitutions, making this journey livable, sustainable, and enjoyable with GREAT food.

Cont.

Introduction

desire to stop eating normal food and no desire to exercise (at that time). The first few weeks were difficult but manageable. I was losing weight, I wasn't working out, but dear Lord, there was so much food that I missed eating that I couldn't have because it was so high in points. Then it happened... I found the "recipe builder" tool, within the WW mobile phone App, that pretty much changed everything.

I immediately realized the full possibilities the tool offered. I bought a cooking magazine from the grocery store, that had a recipe on the cover for a skillet full of baked rolls covered in tons of cheese, marinara sauce, pepperoni and Italian sausage. The type of meal there is NO WAY you could ever eat on Weight Watchers and stay within your points.

I scoured Connect for ingredient swap ideas and even came up with a few ideas of my own. I started swapping out regular cheese for fat free cheese and mixed in some plain yogurt for added creaminess. I adjusted spice amounts, checked how much wine I could cut with water to reduce the points and still taste it in a sauce. I tried getting as creative as I possibly could to make the skillet as low fat and low calorie as possible. Each time I did that with a new recipe, it became more and more fun, like challenging myself to solve a difficult puzzle. Now I can look at almost any recipe and think of ways to almost immediately start cutting the calories, while retaining the flavor.

Now, I absolutely LOVE doing this. I wake up every day, genuinely looking forward to "what am I going to try and make today?" I love logging in to the WW mobile app to check and see if there's anyone that needs a question answered, or needs help with a recipe... I love getting tagged by people who are looking for help.

After being stuck in a house, changing diapers, vacuuming, or being a taxi all day... getting to interact with adults who value you and want to chat, even if it's digitally, is such a relief.

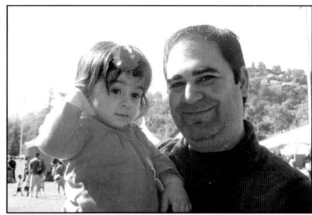

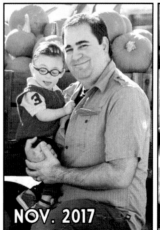

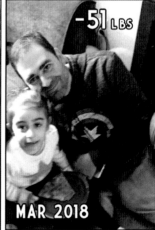

I started Weight Watchers on December 1st, 2017.
I reached my initial goal weight of -51lbs in 3.5 months.
All my weight loss was 100% from changing my cooking habits,
not so much as one moment of intentional exercise.

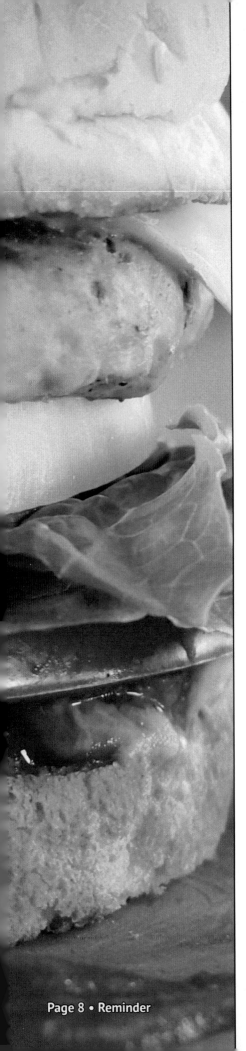

Important Reminder

Just a reminder: Unfortunately, I am unable to include some of the companion recipes that are referenced (or referred to) in this book. As a 'self-publishing' author on Amazon, this publication/cookbook is subject to page constraints. These recipes can be found in my Cookbooks, Volumes 1 & 2.

The most obvious omission is that I am unable to include the 10 pages of meat seasoning mixes, from Cookbook 1, into this Cookbook. There are also a few dressings that are used later in this book, which have their recipes in Cookbook Volume 2 (Hummus, Tartar Sauce, Roasted Garlic & Onion dressing and my Blue Cheese dressing).

There are 2 options for you to easily gain access to the recipes that are referenced.

1. You can view and download both of my prior 2 Cookbooks on my website, in their entirety, for FREE, at: *www.theguiltfreegourmet.net*
2. Both of my other Cookbooks are available on Amazon.

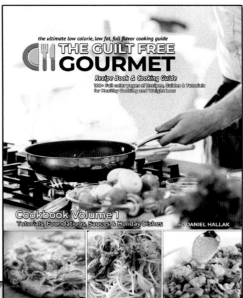

The Guilt Free Gourmet Cookbook Volume 1
- Guides & Tutorials
- Ingredient Swaps
- Meat Seasoning Recipes
- Foundation Recipes
- Sauces
- Holiday Dishes

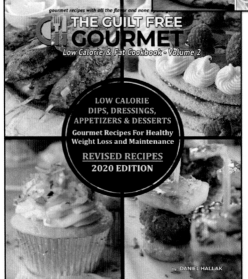

The Guilt Free Gourmet Cookbook Volume 2
- Dips & Spreads
- Salad Dressings
- Gourmet Appetizers
- Gourmet Cupcakes & Cakes

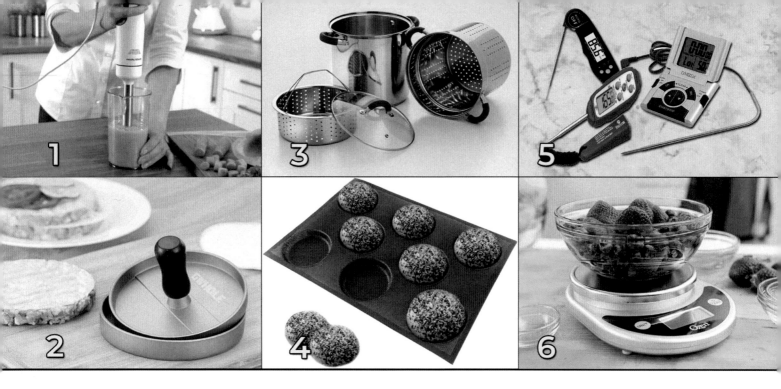

For most of you folks that cook a lot and have spent years trying new things in the kitchen, these Gadgets & Gizmos are nothing new to you. But this particular page is directed more towards people who aren't as comfortable in the kitchen yet and what some of the gadgets are that I use a lot, while making the various recipes in this book.

1. Immersion Blender

YOU NEED THIS IN YOUR LIFE! It's essentially a small blender at the end of a stick. It is used in a few of the dressings in this book, but is used EXTENSIVELY in a ton of the sauces in Cookbooks 1 & 2. You can also use a regular blender, but it takes up a lot more counterspace. You can purchase an inexpensive immersion blender at Target or Walmart.

2. Hamburger Patty Press/Form

Yes... you can form patties individually in your palm. You can also use a candle to cook your dinner, but why would you? When I decided to start making burgers for this book, I broke down and bought a cheap $10 plastic from Amazon and booooy was it worth it. You can get more expensive ones, but I made every burger in this book with a cheap plastic one. I recommend one with a 4.25" diameter. It makes all of your burgers into perfectly shaped patties that are much more visually appealing.

3. Stock Pot with Steamer Inserts

This sounds like something that would be crazy expensive, but I've seen them at Ross and Marshalls for $20-$30. They are so worth it. I use the deep insert to steam cakes inside of a Corningware ceramic round dish, as well as using it to steam my Weight Watchers friendly Tamales (in Cookbook 1). In this book, you use a steamer insert to make the steamed burger buns for my Bahn Mi burgers. You can also use a simple steamer basket that sits over a pot of boiling water. You'll just have to make the buns in multiple batches, rather than all at once.

4. Silicone Burger Bun Mold

If you're going to attempt to make my low point hamburger buns recipe, I highly recommend purchasing a hamburger bun mold. I bought a relatively inexpensive from Amazon. The mold that I purchased is a rubber silicone mold, covered in tiny little perforations, so that no part of the buns burn. The pan that I bought is 17" x 12". The cavities for the buns are 4" across and 1.5" deep. The mold is bendy, so place it on a sheet pan when you actually bake with it.

5. Kitchen Thermometer

First off... you don't need an expensive one. I have a cheap $20 one that I got at Target a few years back. Why do you need one of these? Well... you kind of do and you kind of don't. It depends. IF you plan on making the Yeast Burger Buns (recipe in the 'bonus recipes' section), you have to add water to the yeast that is in an EXACT temperature range. There is no 'add warm water'... the water has to be exactly between 100 and 110 degrees, or your yeast won't proof right. Can you use 'Instant Yeast'? Yes. I don't use it, so my recipe uses 'Active Dry Yeast', which requires 'proofing'. You could definitely use Instant Yeast, but adjust my recipe accordingly.

6. Digital Kitchen Scale

This... is... esseeeential. So many of my burger and sandwich recipes depend upon you weighing cheese or bread, in grams. For instance, if you purchase 4 'Point' burger buns, simply scoop out a little bit of bread from the top bun, then weigh your buns, in 'grams'. You've just made a 3 point bun, by weight. Having a kitchen scale is extremely important for cooking in WW.

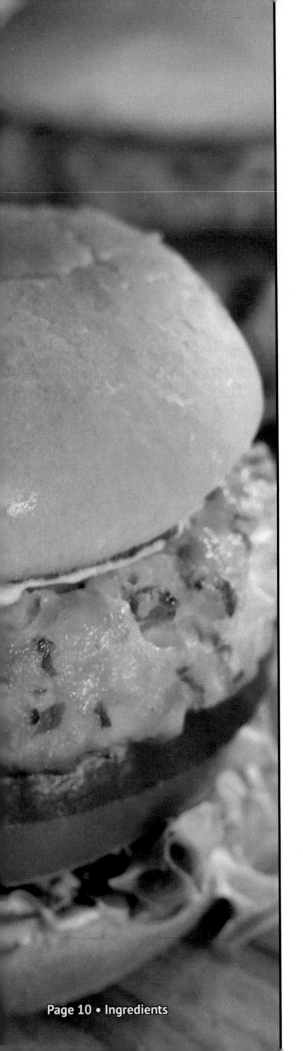

Important Ingredients

Retrain Your Brain

One of the biggest motivations that I have, when making my recipes, is the fun challenge to make them as low in calories and 'Points' as possible, while still keeping a regular, satisfying portion size. These following pages highlight a few of the key ingredients that I feel need to be noted.

99% vs. 93% Ground Turkey & 95% Ground Beef

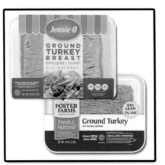

Here's the deal. For you folks that aren't in Weight Watchers and don't care about 'Points', feel free to use 93% fat free ground turkey or extra lean ground beef in ANY of my recipes. The reason that I use 99% fat free ground turkey in my recipes is a Weight Watcher's 'Points' thing. For all of my burger recipes, I used 99% fat free ground turkey. I have developed seasoning mixes and cooking methods that actually make it pretty danged good. Because "Low Points" is my thing… I used it in my recipes, and really liked ALL of my burgers. They are awesome. However, in my own personal time, I use 93%. From the day that I started Weight Watchers, I have ALWAYS counted 93% ground turkey as a "Zero Point Food". That's my own personal thing. If you want to use 99%, awesome. If you want to use 93%, sweet. If you are just here to cook and eat delicious, healthier burgers and don't care about Weight Watchers? Use Beef. Use my recipes as a template and customize them.

Not All Chili Powders Are Created Equal!!!

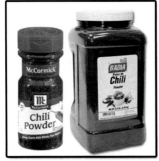

Take It Easy, Don't Burn Your Face Off!

Until recently, I always purchased the least expensive spices I could find… I'm on a budget. My spices were the generic brands from the dollar store and walmart. I recently got a more 'popular' spice brand of Chili Powder than I normally purchase… and MY FACE IS ON FIRE. So remember folks… when a recipe calls for chili powder, different brands have different spice levels. Try using a little less than the recipe calls for, then add more, to taste. This is especially important in recipes that use a decent amount of it, such as my red enchilada sauce and my ground turkey chorizo. You can always add MORE, to taste.

Sugar Free Syrup Instead Of Honey

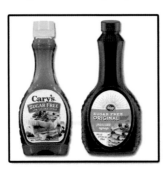

Leave The Food Snobbery At Home

In almost all circumstances, I swap out honey with sugar free pancake syrup (maple flavored) in all my recipes. It's sweet, it's thick, it fills the role I want, while cutting a TON of calories from a sauce or dip. My teriyaki sauce, BBQ sauce, chick-fil-a sauce, 'honey' mustard dressing and others recipes rely on it heavily. Some brands, like 'Cary's', let you have more syrup for 0 points than others.

Dairy Free Yogurt Hack

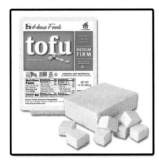

Go Go Gadget, TOFU!

When I first started posting recipes for Greek yogurt based salad dressings and dips, people started asking something I'd never thought of before. What to use instead of Greek yogurt, when you're allergic to dairy? It took a few attempts, but I finally figured it out, Tofu.

Greek yogurt is such a huge building block of so many of my dressings, dips and spreads. A lot of people with allergies automatically assume they can't have a Greek yogurt based recipe. That's not the case. Tofu is readily available at all major grocery stores, inexpensive, and doesn't have a strong flavor (unlike Greek). However, it comes in different levels of firmness. *Firm*, which you can dent a Buick with. *Semi* or *Medium Firm*, which is like a cooled block of cream cheese, then *Silken (or soft)*, which is almost like Plain yogurt.

I blend a 16 ounce block of semi firm tofu with 1/2 cup water, to make a viable replacement for Greek yogurt. It does "tighten" up a bit in the fridge though, so add more water if necessary. If you want that tang that Greek has, add a splash of lemon juice. Does it taste the same as Greek? No, but it's a great alternative, if you have allergies. It works.

Low Calorie, Low 'Point' Sliced Cheese

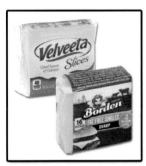

Go Low Or Go Home!!

All of my burgers/sandwiches that call for cheese recommend 'thin sliced' or 'ultra thin sliced' brands of cheese, such as Sargento brand. We're aiming for 40 calories or less per slice, in order to keep it to only adding 1 'Point' per burger. For American cheese, I use 'Velveeta Original' slices, or 'Borden's' Brand, Fat Free Cheddar Slices, which melt like American. Borden's Fat Free can be found at Walmart and some grocery stores. Use it if you can find it. Sargento is in nearly every grocery store. Also... you can go to the deli counter in your store and ask them to cut ANY type of cheese into slices for you. Tell them to cut it AS THIN AS POSSIBLE. Then take it home and weigh the slices in grams. Use the App's ingredient database to find the points for your cheese.

Flavored Cooking Sprays Instead of Oil

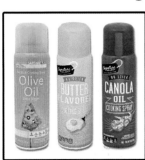

Obvious, but deserves a shout-out

One of the things you'll have to get used to is the idea of using cooking spray, rather than oil, in my recipes. It cuts a ton of calories. Not all brands are created equal though. Some brands let you use only 4 or 5 seconds of spray before they add points. Others let you coat a Buick for 0 points. I typically use generic 'store brands', as they allow you to have more for 0.

Low Calorie, Low 'Point' Bread & Buns

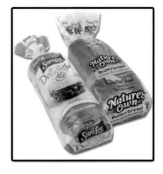

Where To Find It

Choosing low calorie options for your burger's bread or buns is one of those compromises that you are going to decide to make, if you want to continue cutting calories and points. Ask yourself, what would make you feel better, having a giant sized burger bun with 300 calories, or having a smaller sized bun, that'll help you lose weight and still have a burger. Every calorie that you cut, adds up. Saving 150 calories from a bun, 50 calories from the 'lighter' cheese, 60 calories from my ketchup, etc, etc, etc.

To take full advantage of these burger recipes, you'll want to cut the calories and 'Points' from the bread as well. So... where do you find low calorie/Point bread and buns? It's simple.

There are a LOT of options for low 'Point' bread and buns. Lets start with sliced bread. The easiest to find in grocery stores is "Sara Lee 'delightful' 45 calorie bread". It's 1 Point per slice. Sara Lee has whole wheat, multigrain, and white bread versions, though the white bread is harder to find. I usually use the whole wheat. "Nature's Own: Butterbread" is a great tasting sliced white bread that's 1 Point for 1 slice, 3 points for 2 slices. There are tons of different low calorie/Point bread options. You can find extensive lists in a simple google search for "weight watchers friendly bread".

Low Point Burger Buns.... of course there are specific brands of lower point buns. Some people use 'Sandwich Thins', some use 'Light' English muffins, or even wraps. There ARE brands of low point burger buns, same thing, google search for a WW-friendly list of brands and then check your local stores. However... rather than list them all, I'm going to tell you a simple hack you can do with generic store brand buns.

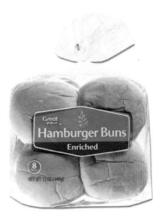

Go to your grocery store and find smaller sized 'old-school' burger buns, look for ones that are 120 or 130 calories per bun. THOSE will scan for either 3 or 4 points. If you only find 4 point buns... buy them.

When you get them home, bust out your kitchen scale and weigh one of the buns, in grams. Scan the bag in the WW app, to pull it up in the ingredient database. Now... the hack.

Scoop a little bit of bread out from the top bun, the 'domed' bun. Now, weigh the bun again, in grams. There is a heck of a good chance that you have just removed enough bread, with that one scoop, to turn your 4 point bun, into a 3 point bun, by weight. Grats... you just made a 3 point burger bun.

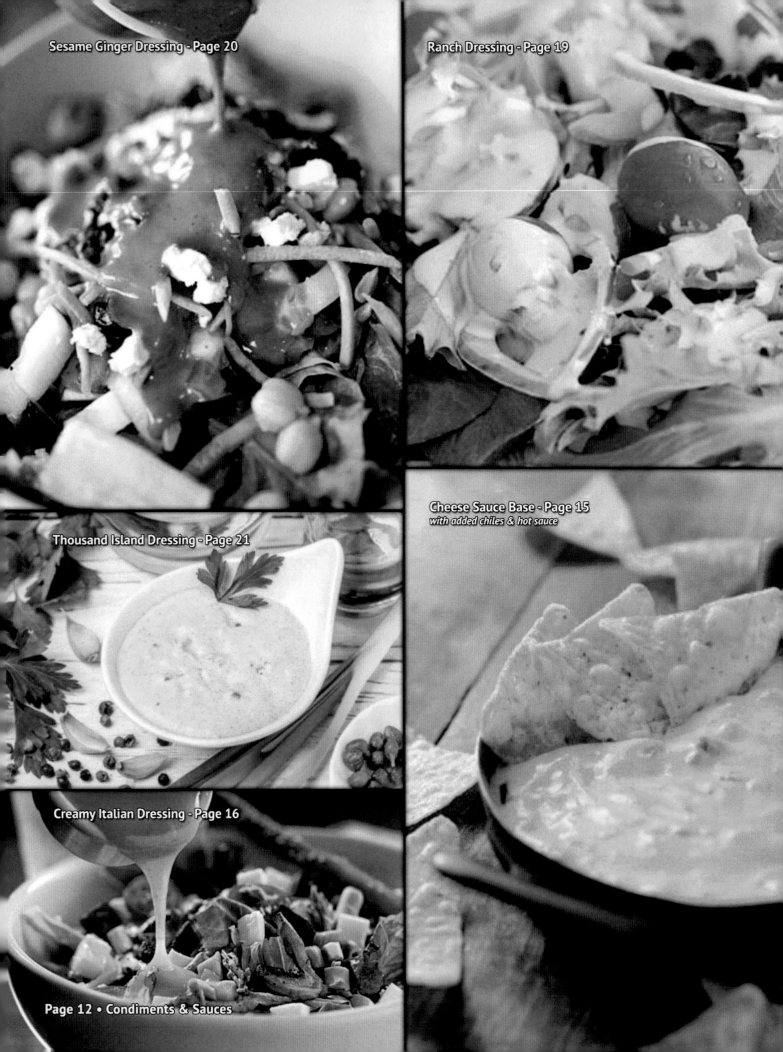

Sesame Ginger Dressing - Page 20

Ranch Dressing - Page 19

Thousand Island Dressing - Page 21

Cheese Sauce Base - Page 15
with added chiles & hot sauce

Creamy Italian Dressing - Page 16

Condiments, Dressings & Spreads

A compilation of the dressings, spreads, sauces & dips used in this book's recipes.
Well, most of them. Blue Cheese Dressing, Hummus, Roasted Garlic & Onion Dressing and Tartar Sauce are in Cookbook 2.

5 Minute Marinara ·············· Pg. 14
Asian Chili Aioli ················ Pg. 14
Asian Orange Sauce & Glaze ······ Pg. 14
BBQ Sauce ··················· Pg. 14
Bruschetta ··················· Pg. 15
Buffalo Sauce ················· Pg. 15
Cheese Sauce ················· Pg. 15
Chick Fil A copycat ············· Pg. 15
Classic Coleslaw Dressing ········· Pg. 16
Creamy Italian Dressing ·········· Pg. 16
Creole Remoulade ·············· Pg. 16
Dark Cherry Sauce ·············· Pg. 16
Dijon Vinaigrette ··············· Pg. 17
Enchilada Sauce ··············· Pg. 17
Garlic Pepper Aioli ············· Pg. 17
Katsu Sauce ·················· Pg. 17
Ketchup ····················· Pg. 18
Lemon White Wine Aioli ·········· Pg. 18
Mango Chili Sauce ·············· Pg. 18
Maple Mustard Spread ··········· Pg. 18
Mayonnaise Substitute ··········· Pg. 19
Mustard Beer Spread ············ Pg. 19
Ranch Dressing ················ Pg. 19
Rice Wine Dressing ············· Pg. 19
Roasted Garlic Mustard Spread ···· Pg. 20
Sesame Ginger Dressing ·········· Pg. 20
Smoky Red Onion & Bacon Jam ···· Pg. 20
Teriyaki Sauce ················ Pg. 21
Thousand Island Dressing ········· Pg. 21
*** Tips & Suggestions ··········· Pg. 21

1. Aside from these dressings, spreads and dips, there are 20 more in Cookbook 2, such as:
Carrot Ginger, Catalina, Caesar, Creamy Chipotle, Roasted Garlic & Onion, Blue Cheese, French, and more.

2. Some of the Greek yogurt based Dressings will "tighten up" a bit more as they rest in the fridge. If they get too thick, simply stir in a little water to thin them out to your desired consistency.

3. Also: If you have allergies to dairy, you can substitute Silken Tofu in place of the Greek yogurt. The taste will be sliiiiiightly different, but it will still work.

5 MINUTE MARINARA SAUCE

This is a VERY fast, small batch Marinara sauce that mixes together in 5 minutes. Leave the Italian food snobbery at home.

Serving Info.:
Yield: 1 cup
Serving Size: 1/4 cup
Servings: 4

Points:

	G	B	P
1 serving =	0	0	0
2 servings =	0	0	0
3 servings =	0	0	0
4 servings =	0	0	0

Ingredients:

- 1 cup tomato sauce
- 1 Tbsp red wine**
- 1/2 tsp garlic powder
- 1/2 tsp onion powder
- 1/4 tsp dried basil
- 1/4 tsp italian seasoning
- 1/2 to 1 tsp 0 point sweetener o' choice, to taste.
- 1/4 tsp salt
- 1/4 tsp pepper

Directions:

1 Bring to a low simmer for 5 minutes. Done.

- If you don't want to use red wine, you can replace it with 1 Tbsp red wine vinegar.
- The sweetener is optional, I like a slightly sweet sauce.
- I don't have time to simmer a sauce for hours. I haz toddlerz.
- I apologize to all of the Italian Nonas, that are marching to my house with torches, pitchforks, and cast iron skillets.

ASIAN CHILI AIOLI

A creamy and spicy blend of Greek yogurt, light mayonnaise sesame oil and Asian garlic chili sauce.

Serving Info.:
Yield: 1/2 cup
Serving Size: 2 Tbsp
Servings: 4

Points:

	G	B	P
1 serving =	0	0	0
2 servings =	0	0	0
3 servings =	0	0	0
4 servings =	0	0	0

Ingredients:

- 2-1/2 Tbsp plain fat free Greek yogurt
- 1 tsp light mayonnaise
- 2 tsp reduced sodium soy sauce
- 2 tsp lemon juice
- 1-2 tsp Asian chili sauce (see notes)
- 1/4 tsp sesame oil
- 1/4 tsp pepper

Directions:

1 Mix all of the ingredients together, till creamy and well blended. Done.

- Asian chili sauce can be found in the Asian food aisle at the grocery store. Typically located by the soy sauce. I used Huy Fong Foods brand garlic chili sauce. They're the same folks that make Sriracha chili sauce.
- This is a small batch sauce, because it's intended to be used to spread on hamburger buns for my Orange Chicken sandwich.

ASIAN 'PANDA' ORANGE SAUCE/GLAZE

This sauce & glaze is a low calorie mashup of Panda's Orange chicken sauce and the sauce from General Tso's chicken.

Serving Info.:
Yield: 1/2 cup
Serving Size: 1/2 cup
Servings: *varies (see notes)*

Points:

	G	B	P
1 serving =	0	0	0
2 servings =	1	1	1
3 servings =	1	1	1
4 servings =	1	1	1

Ingredients:

- 1/4 cup orange juice, some pulp.
- 1 Tbsp orange zest, finely chopped
- 3 Tbsp reduced sodium soy sauce
- 4 Tbsp 0 point sweetener o' choice
- 2 medium garlic cloves, finely chopped
- 1 tsp finely chopped ginger
- 1/8 tsp red pepper flakes, or more to taste.
- 1 Tbsp sugar free syrup (pancake syrup)
- 1/4 tsp pepper
- 1-1/2 tsp cornstarch, dissolved with 2 Tbsp water.
- (optional) 1 tsp toasted sesame seeds, for garnish.

Directions:

1 Bring all of the ingredients to a boil, over medium heat.
2 Simmer for 2-3 minutes or until thickened to desired consistency. It will thicken slightly when removed from heat.

- Adding the toasted sesame seeds to garnish your dish is a huge flavor boost. Regular sesame seeds are 1 point for 1 tsp, while TOASTED sesame seeds are 0 points for 1 tsp.
- This makes 1/2 cup of sauce/glaze for 1 point. Points per serving will be completely dependent upon your application.

BBQ SAUCE

This is a simplified, small batch version of my regular BBQ sauce, from Cookbook 1. It comes together in under 5 minutes.

Serving Info.:
Yield: 2-1/4 cups
Serving Size: 1/4 cup
Servings: 9

Points:

	G	B	P
1 serving =	0	0	0
2 servings =	0	0	0
3 servings =	0	0	0
4 servings =	0	0	0

Ingredients:

- 15oz canned tomato sauce
- 2 tsp worcestershire sauce
- 1 tsp each of garlic powder, onion powder, black pepper, paprika and molasses.
- 1/2 tsp each of: smoked paprika, ground cumin, dry mustard, salt and liquid smoke (hickory flavor)
- 1/8 to 1/4 tsp chili powder (to taste)
- 2 Tbsp 0 point sweetener o' choice, or... 2 Tbsp 0 point brown sugar substitute.
- 2 Tbsp apple cider vinegar

Directions:

1 Mix everything together, till well combined.
2 Allow to rest for at least 30 minutes for flavors to meld.

Notes:

- Liquid smoke can be found in the condiment aisle at the store, usually.

BRUSCHETTA

This is a small batch recipe used for my 'chicken bruschetta' sandwiches. Think of it as Italian 'pico de gallo'.

Serving Info.:
Yield: 1-1/4 cup
Serving Size: 1/4 cup
Servings: 5

Points:

	G	B	P
1 serving =	0	0	0
2 servings =	1	1	1
3 servings =	1	1	1
4 servings =	1	1	1

Ingredients:

- 1-1/4 large tomato, diced (1 cup diced)
- 1/4 cup fresh basil, loosely packed, finely chopped
- 2 medium cloves garlic, smashed, finely chopped
- 1/2 tsp salt
- 1/4 tsp pepper
- 1/4 tsp 'robust' olive oil
- 1-1/2 tsp balsamic vinegar

Directions:

1 Mix everything together in a bowl, cover, allow to sit for at least 30 minutes.

- Some recipes call for adding diced onion, mine doesn't. Feel free to add it if you'd like. It will bulk up the dish and add servings, but will give it a 'sharper' flavor, due to the raw onion.

BUFFALO SAUCE

A quick and easy, small batch dipping sauce, that you can make with any hot pepper sauce that you prefer.

Serving Info.:
Yield: 1 cup
Serving Size: 1/4 cup
Servings: 4

Points:

	G	B	P
1 serving =	0	0	0
2 servings =	0	0	0
3 servings =	0	0	0
4 servings =	0	0	0

Ingredients:

- 3/4 cup red pepper sauce. I used Frank's Red Hot cayenne pepper sauce.
- 2 Tbsp white vinegar
- 1/2 tsp garlic powder
- 2 tsp worcestershire sauce
- 1/8 tsp salt
- 2 Tbsp plain fat free Greek yogurt

Directions:

1 Mix everything together till smooth, done.

- This is a small batch recipe, intended to be used as a drizzled sauce on my buffalo chicken sandwich. If you'd like it to have a thicker consistency, you can either:
  * Blue/Purple Plan: Mix in a little more Greek yogurt.
  * All Plans: In a small pot, heat the first 5 ingredients with 1-1/2 tsp cornstarch, till boiling. Boil for 2-3 minutes. Remove from heat. When the sauce cools to room temperature and thickens, stir in the Greek.

CHEESE SAUCE

A small batch of cheese sauce, that's used to 'sauce' a pot of my Macaroni & Cheese. Use it to 'sauce' a small pot of cooked pasta.

Serving Info.:
Yield: 2/3 cup
Serving Size: 2/3 cup
Servings: 1

Points:

	G	B	P
Entire Batch =	4	4	4

I'm only putting 1 serving, because it's intended use is for a pot of mac n cheese. If you use it for another purpose, adjust the points per serving.

Ingredients:

- 3/4 cup chicken broth
- 2 slices low fat, calorie & 'point' american or cheddar cheese.
- I used Velveeta Originals, I encourge you to use 'Borden's Fat Free Cheddar slices', if you can find them.
- 1/8 tsp salt
- 1/4 tsp ground turmeric (for color)
- 1 Tbsp cornstarch, dissolved in 1 Tbsp water.

Directions:

1 Bring all of the ingredients to a low rolling boil in a small pot, stirring to help the cheese melt. Simmer for 4 minutes. Done.

- These points were calculated with Velveeta. If you use different low point cheese slices, adjust your points.

CHICK-FIL-A COPYCAT SAUCE & DIP

A small batch, revised version of my Chick-Fil-A copycat dip, originally in Cookbook 2.

Serving Info.:
Yield: 1-1/4 cup
Serving Size: 1/4 cup
Servings: 5

Points:

	G	B	P
1 serving =	1	0	0
2 servings =	1	1	1
3 servings =	2	1	1
4 servings =	2	2	2

Ingredients:

- 1/2 cup plain fat free Greek yogurt
- 1 Tbsp light mayonnaise
- 2 Tbsp yellow mustard
- 1 Tbsp dijon mustard
- 1 Tbsp lemon juice
- 1/8 tsp ground turmeric (optional, for color)
- 1/4 tsp dry mustard
- 3 Tbsp sugar free syrup (pancake syrup)
- 1/2 cup tomato sauce
- 1-1/2 Tbsp 0 point sweetener o' choice PLUS 1/4 tsp molasses, or... 1-1/2 Tbsp 0 point brown sugar substitute
- 1/2 tsp worcestershire sauce
- 1/4 tsp garlic powder
- 1/4 tsp onion powder
- 1/2 tsp smoked paprika
- 1 Tbsp apple cider vinegar
- 1/4 tsp black pepper

Directions:

1 Mix everything together till smooth, done.

- We're essentially making a small batch of honey mustard and bbq sauce, then mixing them together with greek and mayo.
- The sugar free syrup replaces the 50 billion points from Honey. The flavor's a bit different from regular, but it's still really good.

CLASSIC COLESLAW DRESSING

A simple, creamy and sweet base for coleslaws and salads. Customize with toasted sesame or poppy seeds... it's a great base.

Serving Info.:
Yield: 2/3 cup
Serving Size: 2/3 cup
Servings: 1

Points:

	G	B	P
Entire Batch	2	1	1

Ingredients:

- 1/2 cup plain fat free Greek yogurt
- 1 Tbsp light mayonnaise
- 2 Tbsp water
- 2 Tbsp apple cider vinegar
- 3 Tbsp 0 point sweetener o' choice
- 1/2 tsp salt
- 1/4 tsp pepper

Directions:

1 Mix everything together till smooth, done.

CREAMY ITALIAN DRESSING

A quick, tasty smaller batch recipe of my copycat Olive Garden Italian dressing. Perfect for traditional and pasta salads.

Serving Info.:
Yield: 1 cup
Serving Size: 1/4 cup
Servings: 4

Points:

	G	B	P
1 serving =	1	0	0
2 servings =	2	1	1
3 servings =	2	1	1
4 servings =	3	1	1

Ingredients:

- 1/2 cup water
- 1-1/2 tsp cornstarch
- 1 large egg yolk***
- 1/4 cup white wine vinegar***
- 1/4 tsp salt
- 1/4 tsp pepper
- 2 tsp lemon juice
- 1 tsp minced garlic
- 1/4 tsp each, dried oregano, basil & parsley
- 1/8 tsp red pepper flakes
- 1 tsp worcestershire sauce
- 1 tsp light mayonnaise
- 1 tsp 0 point sweetener o' choice
- 2-1/2 Tbsp plain fat free Greek yogurt
- 4 tsp Kraft (or other brand) reduced fat, grated parmesan topping.

Directions:

1 Mix and heat the water, cornstarch and yolk in a small pot to a low boil. Simmer and stir for 3 minutes, set aside.
2 Use a small blender or immersion blender to blend ALL the ingredients together, till smooth.
3 Season with additional salt and pepper, if needed.

- You can replace the egg yolk with 1 Tbsp dijon mustard. It'll change the flavor a bit, but lowers the points by 2, for Greenies.
- It's ok that the egg yolk cooks a bit, it all gets blended.

CREOLE REMOULADE

Well, actually, it's my low point recipe for the Outback Steakhouse Bloomin' Onion sauce, but spiced up with some Cajun seasonings.

Serving Info.:
Yield: 1/2 cup
Serving Size: 2 Tbsp
Servings: 4

Points:

	G	B	P
1 serving =	0	0	0
2 servings =	1	1	1
3 servings =	1	1	1
4 servings =	1	1	1

Ingredients:

- 2-1/2 Tbsp plain fat free Greek yogurt
- 1 Tbsp light mayonnaise
- 1 Tbsp store bought "prepared" horseradish sauce
- 1 Tbsp stone ground mustard
- 1 Tbsp apple cider vinegar
- 1 to 2 tsp hot sauce, to taste
- 1/4 tsp garlic powder
- 1/2 tsp smoked paprika
- 1 Tbsp store bought, no sugar added ketchup... or use my Ketchup recipe if you have some on hand.
- 1 tsp lemon juice
- 1/8 tsp salt
- 1/8 tsp pepper
- 1/2 to 1 tsp cajun seasoning, to taste

Directions:

1 Mix everything together till smooth, done.

- The Outback Steakhouse Bloomin' Onion sauce is really just a mix of smoky ketchup, cocktail sauce and mustard. In this recipe I'm making it "Cajun", by adding the hot sauce and cajun seasoning. You can find it in the spice aisle.

DARK CHERRY SAUCE

This sauce is used in my Thanksgiving burger, because cranberries were out of season. I'll honestly never make regular cranberry sauce again, because of how amazing this is.

Serving Info.:
Yield: 1/2 cup
Serving Size: 2 Tbsp
Servings: 4

Points:

	G	B	P
1 serving =	0	0	0
2 servings =	0	0	0
3 servings =	0	0	0
4 servings =	0	0	0

Ingredients:

- 1 cup fresh dark 'sweet' cherries, halved, pits removed.
- 1/2 cup water
- 2 Tbsp 0 point sweetener o' choice PLUS 1/4 tsp molasses, or... 2 Tbsp 0 point brown sugar substitute.
- 1/8 tsp each, ground cinnamon, ginger & nutmeg
- 2 tsp lemon juice
- 1 tsp cornstarch, dissolved with 1 Tbsp water.

Directions:

1 Slice the cherries in half and remove the pits.
2 Add all of the ingredients together, EXCEPT FOR the cornstarch. Bring to a low boil, in a small pot, for 10 minutes.
3 Mash up the cherries, in the pot. Add the cornstarch mixture and simmer for 3 minutes. Set aside to cool.

DIJON VINAIGRETTE

This recipe will make a 0 point dressing that yields juuuuust enough vinaigrette to dress a good sized salad for 2 people.

Serving Info.:
Yield: 1/4 cup
Serving Size: 1/4 cup
Servings: 1

Points:	G	B	P
1 serving =	0	0	0
2 servings =	0	0	0
3 servings =	0	0	0
4 servings =	0	0	0

Ingredients:

- 2-1/2 Tbsp plain fat free Greek yogurt
- 1 Tbsp dijon mustard
- 1/4 tsp olive oil
- 2 tsp white wine vinegar
- 1/8 tsp pepper
- 1/8 tsp salt

Directions:

1 Mix everything together till smooth, done.

- This is one of my few recipes I will ever post for a sauce or dressing, that doesn't have a good sized serving. This was made to 'dress' the arugala for my French Bistro Burger recipe.

ENCHILADA SAUCE - red

This is a revised, small batch version of my enchilada sauce, that was first presented in Cookbook 1. This is used for my enchilada burger. This quick recipe comes together in minutes.

Serving Info.:
Yield: 3 cups
Serving Size: 1/4 cup
Servings: 12

Points:	G	B	P
1 serving =	0	0	0
2 servings =	0	0	0
3 servings =	0	0	0
4 servings =	0	0	0

Ingredients:

- 15oz tomato sauce
- 1-1/2 cups fat free chicken broth
- 1-1/2 tsp garlic powder
- 1-1/2 tsp onion powder
- 1-1/2 tsp ground cumin
- 1 to 2 tsp chili powder, to taste.
- 1/4 tsp salt

Directions:

1 Mix everything together in a small pot and bring to a boil.
2 Reduce heat to a low simmer, cook for 5 minutes. Done.

- Different brands of chili powder have different levels of spiciness. Adjust the spice to your own tastes. You don't want to burn your face off. Start with 1 tsp, then add more if needed.
- For a smokier flavor, add a little bit of McCormick's chipotle chili powder and some smoked paprika.

GARLIC & BLACK PEPPER AIOLI

This is a deliiiiicious spread of Greek yogurt, garlic, mayo, parmesan and black pepper. It's tasty AND keeps vampires at bay.

Serving Info.:
Yield: 2/3 cup
Serving Size: 2 Tbsp
Servings: 5

Points:	G	B	P
1 serving =	0	0	0
2 servings =	1	0	0
3 servings =	1	1	1
4 servings =	2	1	1

Ingredients:

- 1/2 cup fat free plain Greek yogurt
- 1 Tbsp light mayonnaise
- 2 Tbsp lemon juice
- 2 Tbsp water
- 2 garlic cloves, crushed, minced
- 1-1/2 tsp Kraft (or other brand) reduced fat grated parmesan topping.
- 1/4 tsp garlic powder
- 1/2 tsp black pepper
- 1/2 tsp salt

Directions:

1 Mix everything together till smooth, done.

- Don't have fresh garlic? Add an extra 1/2 tsp garlic powder.
- Food snobbie and don't want to use reduced fat parmesan topping? No problem, use the real stuff. I have toddlers... I'm not buying "real" parmesan for their spaghetti and pizza. lol
- If you use a differnt kind of parmesan cheese, adjust your points.

KATSU SAUCE

Common in Japanese steak houses, this thick, savory sauce is a blend of tomato and soy sauce, worcestershire and spices.

Serving Info.:
Yield: 1 cup
Serving Size: 1/4 cup
Servings: 4

Points:	G	B	P
1 serving =	0	0	0
2 servings =	1	1	1
3 servings =	1	1	1
4 servings =	1	1	1

Ingredients:

- 1/2 cup tomato sauce
- 2 Tbsp + 1 tsp worcestershire sauce
- 2-1/2 Tbsp low sodium soy sauce
- 3 Tbsp rice wine vinegar
- 1-1/2 tsp cornstarch dissolved in 1 Tbsp water
- 1/2 tsp garlic powder
- 1/2 tsp onion powder
- 1/2 tsp ground ginger
- 1/8 tsp celery salt**
- 1/4 tsp pepper
- 2 Tbsp 0 point sweetener o' choice

Directions:

1 Stir all of the ingredients together in a small pot, till smooth. Then bring to a boil over medium heat.
2 Cook at a rolling boil for 1 minute, then turn off heat. Pour into a cup and cool to room temperature. Done.

- Don't want to buy celery salt just to use that tiny amount? Just use regular salt, I won't tell.

KETCHUP

A simplified and smaller batch recipe for my original spiced ketchup from Cookbook 2.

Serving Info.:
Yield: 1-1/4 cup
Serving Size: 1/4 cup
Servings: 5

Points:

	G	B	P
1 serving =	0	0	0
2 servings =	0	0	0
3 servings =	1	1	1
4 servings =	1	1	1

Ingredients:

- 1 cup canned, unsalted tomato sauce
- 2 Tbsp unsalted tomato paste
- 1 Tbsp apple cider vinegar
- 1 Tbsp lemon juice
- 1 tsp worcestershire sauce
- 1/2 tsp celery salt
- 1/4 tsp each, onion powder, garlic powder, pepper
- 1 Tbsp 0 point sweetener o' choice

Directions:

1 Mix everything together till smooth, done.

- You can replace the celery salt with regular salt, but it will not have that nice, savory flavor.
- If you don't have apple cider vinegar, distilled white vinegar works fine too.
- You don't haaaave to make my ketchup, feel free to use any brand you want. But, homemade tastes better. Plus, you can control what goes into your food. Also, mine's lower in total points, fat and calories.

LEMON & WHITE WINE AIOLI

This small batch, creamy Greek & Mayo spread, is used on my salmon burgers. However, it's also a great substitute for tartar sauce.

Serving Info.:
Yield: 1 cup
Serving Size: 1/4 cup
Servings: 4

Points:

	G	B	P
1 serving =	1	0	0
2 servings =	2	1	1
3 servings =	2	1	1
4 servings =	3	1	1

Ingredients:

- 3/4 cup plain fat free Greek yogurt
- 1 Tbsp light mayonnaise
- 1 Tbsp dijon mustard
- 1 Tbsp white wine (chardonnay)
- 1 tsp finely chopped fresh dill
- 2 tsp lemon juice
- 1/2 tsp finely chopped lemon zest
- 1/4 tsp salt
- 1/8 tsp pepper

Directions:

1 Mix everything together till smooth, done.

- This was made to be used for my salmon burger, but it would be just as delicious used with any seafood dish, or even in place of traditional tartar sauce.

MANGO CHILI SAUCE

This versatile and simple recipe can be easily customized to use any fruit that you have on hand, simply replace the mango.

Serving Info.:
Yield: 1-1/4 cup
Serving Size: 1/4 cup
Servings: 5

Points:

	G	B	P
1 serving =	0	0	0
2 servings =	0	0	0
3 servings =	0	0	0
4 servings =	0	0	0

Ingredients:

- 1 good sized mango, pureed. Skin and pit removed. You end up with between 1 to 1-1/4 cups of puree.
- 1 Tbsp Asian garlic chili sauce, such as Huy Fong brand, from the Sriracha folks.
- 1 tsp 0 point sweetener o' choice
- 1/4 tsp salt

Directions:

1 Mix everything together till smooth, done.

Notes:

- I suck at cutting mangos. If your local store has ready-cut mango slices in the produce department, snatch those babies up! You can also find them in the frozen food aisle.
- Need to know how to clean and slice a mango? Youtube.
- This is highly customizable. Don't like mango? Puree some peaches or pineapple instead.
- No, Susie, even though it's pureed, this fruit stays 0 points. WW rules state that blended fruit gets points when you DRINK IT... not when you use is as a component of a dish that you eat. So.... next time you drink a smoothie try chewing some bubble gum at the same time. 😆😂🤣

MAPLE MUSTARD DRESSING/SPREAD

This is a SMALL batch, 1/2 cup recipe. It's enough to 'dress' 'a laaaaaaaarge salad, or to be used as a spread on burger buns.

Serving Info.:
Yield: 1/2 cup
Serving Size: 2 Tbsp
Servings: 4

Points:

	G	B	P
1 serving =	0	0	0
2 servings =	0	0	0
3 servings =	0	0	0
4 servings =	0	0	0

Ingredients:

- 2-1/2 Tbsp plain fat free Greek yogurt
- 1 Tbsp dijon mustard
- 3 Tbsp traditional yellow mustard
- 1 Tbsp sugar free maple syrup (pancake syrup)
- 1/2 to 1 tsp 0 point sweetener o' choice (to taste).
- 1 tsp light mayonnaise
- 1 Tbsp lemon juice
- 1/4 tsp black pepper
- dash of hot sauce, to taste (optional).

Directions:

1 Mix everything together till smooth, done.

- Some brands of sugar free/light pancake syrup, allow you to use 2 Tbsp for 0 points. Use as much as you can for 0.
- This is my low point answer to Honey Mustard dressing.

LOW FAT MAYONNAISE SUBSTITUTE

This is a simple little blend of reduced fat light mayonnaise, mixed with a little bit of fat free Greek yogurt. I use it in everything.

Serving Info.:
Yield: 1 cup
Serving Size: 1/4 cup
Servings: 4

Points:	G	B	P
1 serving =	0	0	0
2 servings =	1	1	1
3 servings =	1	1	1
4 servings =	1	1	1

Ingredients:
- 1/2 cup plain fat free Greek yogurt
- 1 Tbsp light mayonnaise
- 1 tsp dijon mustard
- 1/8 tsp salt

Directions:
1 Stir all of the ingredients together till well mixed. Done.

MUSTARD & BEER SPREAD

This small batch recipe was created as a spread for my Oktoberfest burgers. You gotta have beer and mustard, after all.

Serving Info.:
Yield: 1/2 cup
Serving Size: 2 Tbsp
Servings: 4

Points:	G	B	P
1 serving =	0	0	0
2 servings =	0	0	0
3 servings =	0	0	0
4 servings =	0	0	0

Ingredients:
- 2 Tbsp (1oz) Light Beer. Yes.... light beer, deal with it.
- 1 Tbsp dijon mustard
- 2 Tbsp traditional yellow mustard
- 1 Tbsp whole grain, stone ground mustard
- 2 Tbsp fat free plain Greek yogurt
- 1/2 tsp dry mustard powder
- 1/4 tsp salt
- 1/4 tsp pepper
- a dash of hot sauce, to taste (optional)

Directions:
1 Mix everything together, till well combined.
2 Allow 30 minutes for flavors to meld.

- This entire 1/2 cup of dressing, has no points.
- If the beer in this spread, will knock you off your 12-step program... replace it with water. It's still tasty, without the suds.

Oktoberfest Burger, with Mustard & Beer Spread

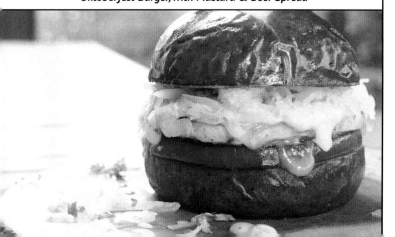

RANCH DRESSING

This is Weight Watchers 101, but new folks are ALWAYS asking how to make quick, easy, low point Ranch dressing. So, here'ya go.

Serving Info.:
Yield: 1 cup
Serving Size: 1/4 cup
Servings: 4

Points:	G	B	P
1 serving =	1	0	0
2 servings =	2	1	1
3 servings =	2	1	1
4 servings =	3	1	1

Ingredients:
- 7/8 cup plain fat free Greek yogurt. It's easy. Measure 1 cup, then scoop out 2 Tablespoons. *(it's a 'points' thing, for Greenies)*
- 1/4 cup plain unsweetened almond milk (or water)
- 1 Tbsp light mayonnaise
- 1-2 tsp Hidden Valley Ranch buttermilk dressing & seasoning mix, to taste. (the powdered stuff, in the little packets)

Directions:
1 Mix everything together till smooth, set aside 30 minutes. Done.

- The 'exact' measurements of the almond milk and Greek yogurt are for the benefit of folks on the Green plan. If you are on Blue or Purple, you can add the full 1 cup of Greek, then use a total of 2 tsp of the dry Ranch mix.

RICE WINE DRESSING

This quick and easy dressing is used in my Asian cabbage 'slaw' that goes onto my crispy orange chicken sandwich.

Serving Info.:
Yield: 1/4 cup
Serving Size: 1/4 cup
Servings: 1

Points:	G	B	P
1 serving =	0	0	0
2 servings =	0	0	0
3 servings =	0	0	0
4 servings =	0	0	0

Ingredients:
- 1-1/2 Tbsp plain fat free Greek yogurt
- 1 Tbsp rice wine vinegar
- 2 Tbsp lemon juice
- 1/4 tsp sesame oil
- 2 tsp 0 point sweetener o' choice
- 1/4 tsp salt
- 1/4 tsp pepper
- (optional) 1 tsp toasted sesame seeds

Directions:
1 Mix everything together till smooth, done.

Notes:
- This is a small batch recipe, intended to lightly dress a large bowl of coleslaw or salad. It is a thin dressing, so it easily coats a large salad, though making a small yield dressing.
- 1 tsp of regular sesame seeds is 1 point. 1 tsp of TOASTED sesame seeds is 0.

ROASTED GARLIC & MUSTARD SPREAD

This is another small batch recipe intended as a spread for my aaaaawesomely delicious, Cuban "Havana Burgers" recipe.

Serving Info.:
Yield: 1/2 cup
Serving Size: 2 Tbsp
Servings: 4

Points:

	G	B	P
1 serving =	0	0	0
2 servings =	1	0	0
3 servings =	1	0	0
4 servings =	1	0	0

Ingredients:

- 4 medium cloves fresh garlic, in their skin.
- cooking spray
- foil paper
- 6 Tbsp fat free plain Greek yogurt
- 2 Tbsp yellow classic mustard
- 1 Tbsp dijon mustard
- 1 tsp light mayonnaise
- 2 to 3 tsp water, to desired consistency
- salt and pepper to taste

Directions:

1 Preheat oven to 375 degrees. Snip the tip off of 1 side from each garlic clove. Put into a foil pouch, spray with cooking spray, then close pouch. Bake for 45 minutes.
2 Let garlic cool for 10 mins. Squeeze roasted garlic out of the skins, then mash with a fork.
3 Mix all ingredients together till smooth, season to taste.

- To make future batches easier, you can always make a larger batch of roasted garlic and freeze the excess, for later.
- Though created for my 'Cuban', you can use it on any sandwich that you make here in the good ol' US of A.... 'muuuurica!

SESAME GINGER DRESSING

This recipe will make JUST ENOUGH, to 'dress' a good sized salad, that can be shared by up to 4 people.

Serving Info.:
Yield: 1/4 cup
Serving Size: 1/4 cup
Servings: 1

Points:

	G	B	P
1 serving =	0	0	0
2 servings =	0	0	0
3 servings =	0	0	0
4 servings =	0	0	0

Ingredients:

- 1 tsp toasted sesame seeds
- 2-1/2 Tbsp plain fat free Greek yogurt
- 1 tsp light mayonnaise
- 1/4 tsp ground ginger
- 1/4 tsp sriracha or other asian chili sauce
- 1-1/4 tsp lime juice
- 1 Tbsp soy sauce
- 1/2 tsp 0 point sweetener o' choice
- 1 tsp powdered peanut butter (leave out, if allergic)
- 1/4 tsp sesame oil
- additional water, for thinning to desired consistency.

Directions:

1 Add plain sesame seeds into a hot pan over medium heat, for 3-4 minutes, till very fragrant. Remove from heat.
2 Mix all of the ingredients together until well combined. Done.

SMOKY RED ONION & BACON JAM

This jam is earth shakingly amazing. It's a low sugar, fat and calorie BACON JAM for goodness sake!! Spread it on everything!

Serving Info.:
Yield: 1-1/2 cup
Serving Size: 1/4 cup
Servings: 6

Points:

	G	B	P
1 serving =	1	1	1
2 servings =	1	1	1
3 servings =	2	2	2
4 servings =	3	3	3

Ingredients:

- 3-4 slices turkey bacon or 'center cut' regular bacon. 4 points worth (see notes)***
- 3.5 to 4 cups red onion, halved and sliced thin.
- 1-1/2 cups beef broth (scan to ensure it's 0 points)
- 2 Tbsp apple cider vinegar
- 1/4 tsp salt
- 1/4 tsp black pepper
- 1 tsp 0 point brown sugar substitute, OR 1 tsp regular sweetener plus 1/4 tsp molasses.
- 1/2 tsp smoked paprika
- 1/2 tsp unsweetened cocoa powder
- 2 tsp balsamic vinegar
- 1-2 Tbsp sugar free syrup (pancake syrup). Scan the brands, some give 1 Tbsp for 0 points, some allow 2 Tbsp.

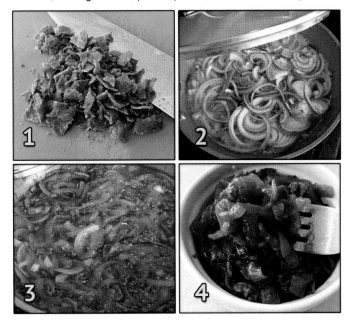

Directions:

1 Cook all of the bacon in a large pan, with cooking spray, till crisp. Remove from pan and chop into small pieces. Set aside.
2 To the same pan, add the sliced red onions, 3/4 cup beef broth, apple cider vinegar, salt, pepper and brown sugar substitute or sweetener and molasses. Bring to a simmer, cover and cook for 15 minutes.
3 After 15 minutes, add the remaining 3/4 cup beef broth, smoked paprika, cocoa powder, balsamic vinegar, syrup and chopped bacon. Cover and simmer on medium-low for another 15 to 20 minutes, or until...
4 ... it resembles a thick jam. Add more salt and pepper, if desired.

NOTES:
- 'Center Cut' bacon is lower in points than regular, fattier bacon. Most brands are virtually identical in points to turkey bacon.

TERIYAKI SAUCE

This sauce is truly awesome and comes together really fast. Is it authentic? No. Is it tasty and does it fit the flavor profile? Yup.

Serving Info.:
Yield: 1 cup
Serving Size: 1/4 cup
Servings: 4

Points:

	G	B	P
1 serving =	0	0	0
2 servings =	0	0	0
3 servings =	0	0	0
4 servings =	0	0	0

Ingredients:

- 3/4 cup water
- 1-1/2 tsp cornstarch
- 2 Tbsp 0 point sweetener o' choice PLUS 1/4 tsp molasses, or... 2 Tbsp 0 point brown sugar substitute.
- 3 Tbsp low sodium soy sauce
- 1 Tbsp sugar free syrup (pancake syrup)
- 1 medium garlic clove, chopped
- 1/4 tsp ground ginger
- 1/8 tsp salt
- 1/8 tsp red pepper flakes (optional)

Directions:

1. Pour the water into a small sauce pot, stir in the cornstarch to dissolve, then add the rest of the ingredients.
2. Bring the sauce to a boil for 4-5 minutes. Remove from heat, cool to room temperature.
3. The sauce will thicken more as it cools. Stir every few minutes as it cools, so that it doesn't get a thin, firm layer on top from the cornstarch.

Notes:

- You can replace the "0 point sweetener o' choice" and the molasses from the recipe and use 2 Tbsp of 0 point brown sugar substitute instead.

THOUSAND ISLAND DRESSING

A quick, simplified and smaller batch recipe for my original Thousand Island dressing from Cookbok 2.

Serving Info.:
Yield: 1-1/4 cup
Serving Size: 1/4 cup
Servings: 5

Points:

	G	B	P
1 serving =	1	0	0
2 servings =	1	0	0
3 servings =	2	1	1
4 servings =	2	1	1

Ingredients:

- 3/4 cup fat free plain Greek yogurt
- 1 Tbsp light mayonnaise
- 3 Tbsp tomato sauce
- 1 tsp lemon juice
- 1/4 cup finely diced onion
- 3 Tbsp dill relish
- 1/2 tsp paprika
- 2 tsp 0 point sweetener o' choice
- 1/2 tsp salt
- 1/4 tsp pepper

Directions:

1. Mix it all together, done.

TIPS & SUGGESTIONS:

- The reason that I use only 2-1/2 Tbsp of plain fat free Greek in most of these recipes, is for the folks on the GREEN plan. Anything over 2-1/2 Tbsp adds points for them.

- *SUGAR FREE SYRUP*: I use sugar free pancake (maple) syrup in my recipes, in place of honey. Primarily because of points, and also for folks with diabetes. Most of my dressings only use 1 Tbsp of it. Most brands only let you have 1 Tbsp for 0 points, though SOME brands allow you to have up to 3 Tbsp for 0 points. Scan the brand that you have, and use what you can.

- *SWEETENERS*: I use sweeteners instead of regular sugar, in everything. Again, there's a lot of diabetic folks in my family, also... points and calories. If you prefer to use regular sugar, do so. Use my recipes as a template. I go into much more detail on sweeteners in the dessert section of Cookbook 2.

- *BROWN SUGAR SUBSTITUTE*: In a lot of my recipes, I mention that for you to "use your 0 point sweetener o' choice' PLUS 1/4 tsp of molasses... or... use 0 point brown sugar substitute." The reason being, that regular brown sugar is simply normal granulated sugar, mixed with a small amount of molasses. By adding a little molasses to sweetener (such as monkfruit, swerve, splenda, etc), you are essentially making brown sugar substitute. I do that because I don't want to purchase an extra type of sweetener. I just have regular, plus a jar of molasses.

- *DAIRY ALLERGIES*: I've mentioned it before, but I'll say it again. If you are allergic to dairy, you can substitute the Greek yogurt in all of my dressings, with a bit of semi-firm tofu, that's blended with some water. Silken tofu is too thin. After blending the tofu/water till it's creamy, I add a splash of lemon juice, just so that it has that little yogurt tang to it. It doesn't taste EXACTLY the same, because believe it or not, it's a bit savory... but it's an easy substitution.

Smoky Red Onion & Bacon Jam - Pg. 20

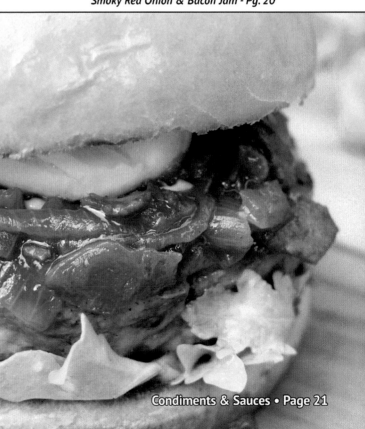

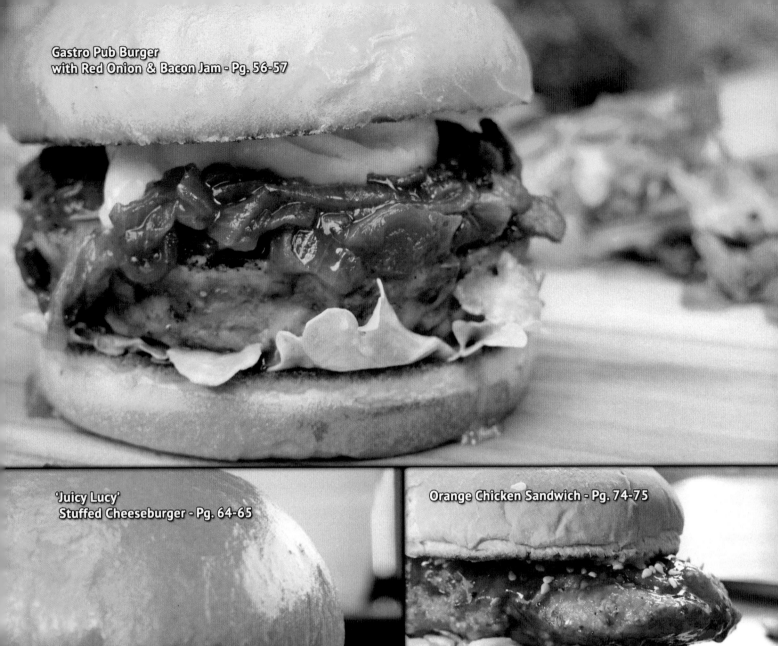

Gastro Pub Burger
with Red Onion & Bacon Jam - Pg. 56-57

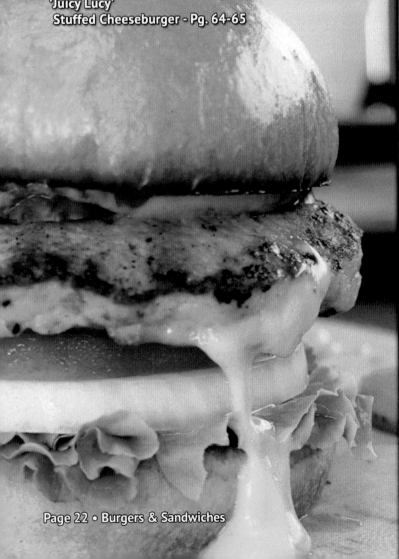

'Juicy Lucy'
Stuffed Cheeseburger - Pg. 64-65

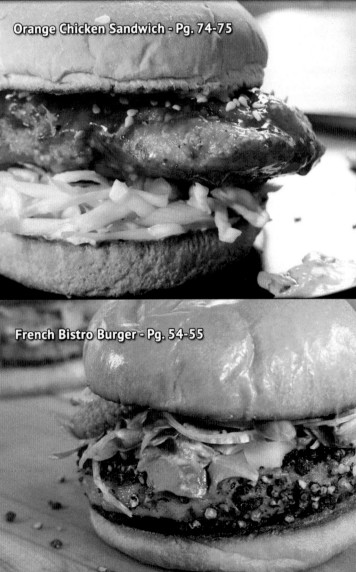

Orange Chicken Sandwich - Pg. 74-75

French Bistro Burger - Pg. 54-55

Burgers & Sandwiches

Tired of having sad and disappointing little slider sized 'burgers' if you want to lose or maintain weight? Want to win over that significant other that gripes about your 'diet food'? Get ready to convert them with 36 GOURMET, low calorie, low fat burgers & sandwiches.

The All American ················ 24-25
Animal Style Cheeseburger ···· 26-27
Bahn Mi ······················· 28-29
Bacon Mac n Cheese ············ 30-31
Big Dan & Junion Dan ·········· 32-33
Blue Cheese & Onion ··········· 34-35
Bruschetta Chicken ············ 36-37
Buffalo Ranch Chicken ········· 38-39
Chicken Club ·················· 40-41
Chicken Cordon Bleu ··········· 42-43
Chicken Parmesan ·············· 44-45
Chick Fil A copycat ··········· 46-47
Cod Sandwich ·················· 48-49
Crispy Fish Sandwich ·········· 50-51
Enchilada Burger ·············· 52-53
French Bistro ················· 54-55
Gastro Pub ···················· 56-57
Green Chili Chorizo ··········· 58-59
Havana (Cuban) ················ 60-61

Bruschetta Chicken Sandwich ... 37-37

Jerk Chicken ·················· 62-63
Juicy Lucy ···················· 64-65
Kafta (Lebanese) ·············· 66-67
Meatloaf Sandwich ············· 68-69
Mushroom & Swiss ·············· 70-71
Oktoberfest (German) ·········· 72-73
Orange Chicken ················ 74-75
Patty Melt ···················· 76-77
Pizza Burger ·················· 78-79
Reuben Burger ················· 80-81
Salmon Burger ················· 82-83
Sausage & Peppers ············· 84-85
Shrimp Po'Boy ················· 86-87
Sloppy Joe ···················· 88-89
Teriyaki ······················ 90-91
Thanksgiving ·················· 92-93
Western Bacon Cheeseburger ····· 94-95
*** Burgers Tips & Suggestions ···· 96-97

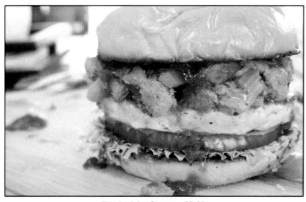

Thanksgiving Burger ... 92-93

*** IMPORTANT ***

The Burgers & Sandwiches in this section DO NOT INCLUDE the points for bread or buns, in the listed points. This is so that you can use whatever bread or bun you would like, be it a high point bun, or a low point bun. Add the points for my recipes, which act as the 'filling' between the bread, to the points for your bread of choice.

Example:

If you are using a 4 point hamburger bun, and my recipe states 1 serving is 2 points... then add the points for your bun to the points for my recipe. That makes your 1 sandwich 6 points. 4 for your bun, 2 for my 'filling'. That same sandwich would be 4 points if you used (2) 1 point pieces of sandwich bread. 2 points for the bread, 2 points for my recipe.

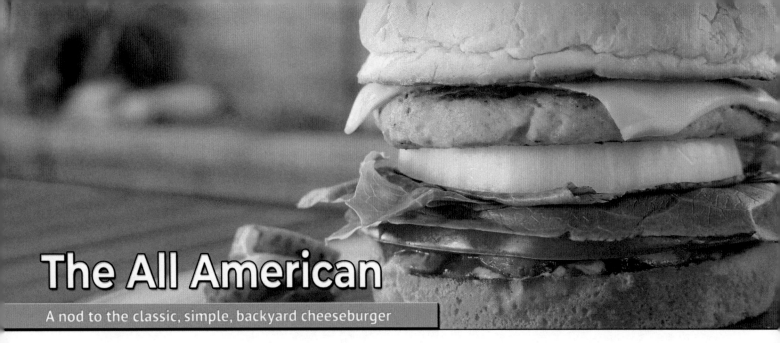

The All American

A nod to the classic, simple, backyard cheeseburger

It occured to me the other day, I've spent months making all of these snazzy and fancy burgers/sandwiches... but I hadn't actually made a simple, old school, classic American cheeseburger. I decided to add this burger, as a throwback to the timeless and simple burgers we all grew up with at family get togethers and backyard pool parties. Nothing fancy... just fresh tomato, lettuce, onion, American cheese, ketchup and mustard, because.... 'Muuuuurica.

Servings Info.:
Yields: 4 burgers
Servings: 4
Serving Size: 1 burger

Points:

1 serving =	G	B	P
1 serving =	3	2	2
2 servings =	6	5	5
3 servings =	9	7	7
4 servings =	12	10	10

(These listed points DO NOT INCLUDE the bun. Use whichever brand buns or bread you want, then add these points. This is what's between the buns)

Ingredients:

Burger Patties
• 1/2 lb batch of my "savory" ground turkey. Recipe in my "Cookbook: Volume 1" on page 30, formed into (4) 2oz patties.

Ketchup:
• 1/2 batch of my low point ketchup recipe. Recipe on page 18.

Additional Toppings:
• 4 slices low point American cheese singles. I used velveeta originals, because everyone can find them.
• Lettuce, any variety.
• 1 tomato, sliced
• 1 onion, sliced into rounds.
• Dill pickle slices
• Yellow mustard

Directions:

1. Prepare a batch of my low point Ketchup, set aside.

2. Slice and prepare the produce, set aside.

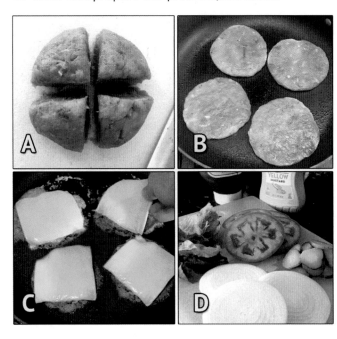

3. **(A)** Divide the 1/2 pound of meat into 4 sections, then heat a pan over medium heat, till droplets of water immediately sizzle in it. **(B)** Spray the pan with cooking spray and fry the patties on medium high heat for 2 minutes, no longer. **(C)** Flip the patties and cover with cheese. Cover with a lid and cook for 2 more minutes. Remove from heat.
(D) Get all of your toppings lined up and ready.

4. Toast your buns (deep squats and Yoga help) and slice your tomatoes. Don't forget to wash and clean your lettuce. We didn't all survive "The 'Rona", just to go and get Norovirus, folks.

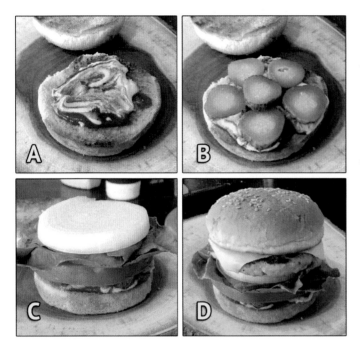

5. To assemble, **(A)** smear some ketchup and yellow mustard on the bottom bun,. **(B)** followed by dill pickle slices. Use as many as you want. **(C)** Place a slice of tomato on top of the pickles, followed by some lettuce and a slice of onion. **(D)** Place a cheeseburger patty on top of the onion, then smear some more ketchup and mustard on the top bun. Done.

NOTES & SUGGESTIONS:

- *POINTS:* The points listed in this recipe assume that you're making 2 to 2.5 ounce, thinner burger patties. That's for 2 reasons: (1) I like thinner patties, I'm eating these... so neener. (2) The thinner patties only add 1 single point for the Green plan folks. If you like meatier burgers and are on Blue/Purple, feel free to make thicker patties, but add 1 minute to the cook time on each side of the patty.
- *LOW POINT CHEESE SLICES:* This recipe has it's points factored with the use of low point "Velveeta Original" slices. There are lower point American cheese slices out there. I prefer "Borden Fat Free Cheddar Slices", but used Velveeta in this recipe, because they are carried at most grocery stores. Use what you want, adjust your points.
- *KETCHUP:* Though my low point Ketchup recipe is "rock star", you obviously can use any brand ketchup that you'd like. If you decide to use store bought ketchup, adjust your points.
  - *ALSO:* I added 1 point for the ketchup onto each burger, though MY ketchup is 0 points for the first 1/4 cup on all 3 plans. In the recipe builder, combining all of the ingredients for all 4 burgers together adds 1 point to each of them. If you are ONLY going to eat one burger.... honestly... just drop the point for your 1 serving. Do what works for you. Unless I am eating 2 of these... I personally wouldn't count the point for my ketchup.

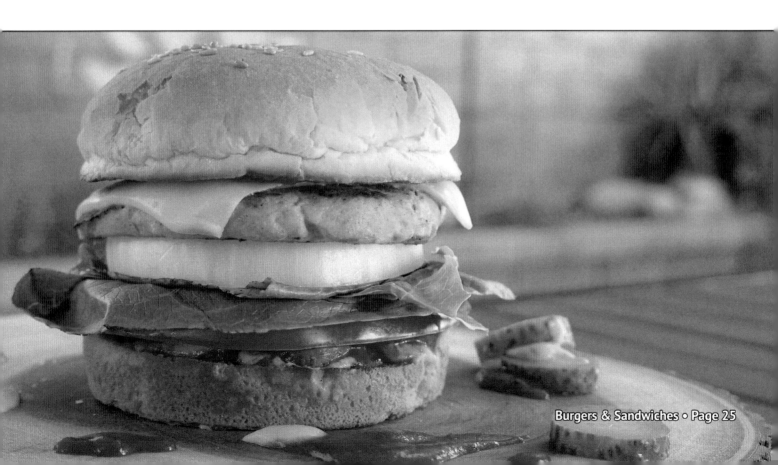

Animal Style Cheeseburger

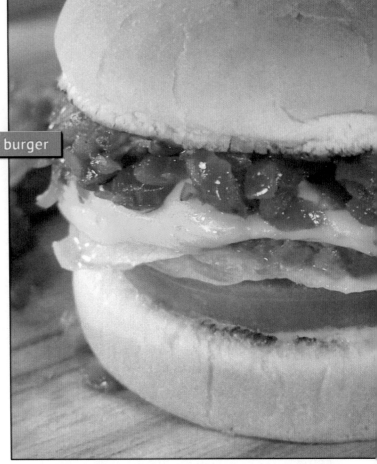

In-n-Out Burger is a West coast institution. Since the beginning of time, the debate has raged on whether or not they make the best fast food burger in the country or not. When you go to In n Out, you can order "secret" menu items, which aren't really secret. The most popular is to order your burger "Animal" style. If you're going to only try In n Out one time... it needs to be an Animal style cheeseburger or Double Double. This recipe is for the single cheeseburger.

Servings Info.:
Yields: 4 burgers
Servings: 4
Serving Size: 1 burger

Points:

	G	B	P
1 serving =	3	2	2
2 servings =	6	4	4
3 servings =	8	5	5
4 servings =	11	7	7

*(These listed points **DO NOT INCLUDE** the bun. Use whichever brand buns or bread you want, then add these points.)*

Ingredients:

Savory Ground Turkey Patties **
- 1/2 lb batch of my Savory Ground Turkey, recipe in my "Cookbook: Volume 1", on page 30.

Thousand Island Dressing:
- Make a batch of my Thousand Island dressing, recipe on page 21.

Caramelized Onions:
- 2 large or 1 jumbo yellow onions, diced small. Seriously, you don't want huge chunks. Take your time and do a fine dice. No arguing, Susie.
- 1/4 tsp salt
- 1/4 tsp pepper
- 1/2 cup water
- 1 Tbsp apple cider vinegar

Additional Ingredients:
- Iceberg lettuce. No whining about it not being fancy. You HAVE to use iceberg.
- 4 slices of low point American cheese (any brand that's 1 point for the first slice. I used Velveeta original in this recipe).
- 4 Tomato slices
- Dill pickle slices
- Kleenex, to wipe your tears of joy, as well as...
- Earplugs, to block out the choir of Angels after your first bite.

Directions:

1. Mix together the ground meat, set aside. Mix together a batch of my Thousand Island dressing, set aside.

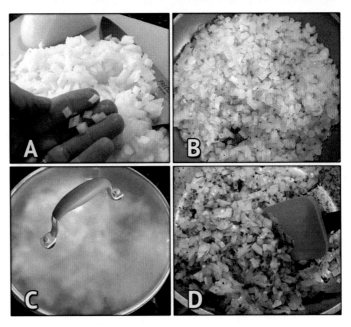

2. (A) I cannot stress this enough. For these In-N-Out burgers, you have to finely dice your onions. **(B)** Heat a pan over medium heat, spray with cooking spray, then add the onions, salt and pepper. Cook for 5 minutes, till the onions begin to sweat. **(C)** Pour the water and vinegar into the pan, stir, then cover. Reduce heat to just under medium. **(D)** Cook, covered, for 15 minutes. Every few minutes remove the lid and stir the onions. If it looks like all the liquid is gone, add another Tablespoon of water, then replace the lid. After 15 minutes, the onions should be nice and caramelized. Keep the lid on, remove pan from heat and set aside.

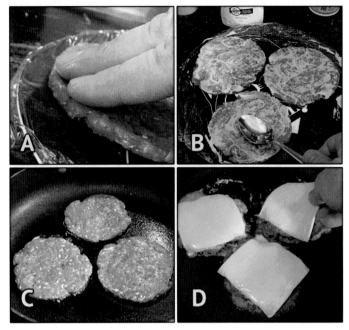

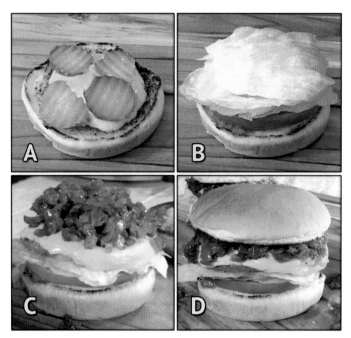

3. **(A)** Form the meat into 4 even patties, these are supposed to be thin patties. After they are formed, press down on them, to make them thinner and wider. Trust me. **(B)** Spread a small amount of yellow mustard across the top of each patty, then start heating up a large pan over medium heat. **(C)** Use cooking spray to cook the patties, mustard side down, for 2 minutes over medium heat. While they are cooking, spread mustard onto the top (raw) side. **(D)** After 2 mins. have passed, flip the patties (mustard-side down again) and place 1 slice of cheese on top. Cook for 2 more minutes. Done.

4. To assemble the burgers, first toast the buns, then **(A)** smear 1 Tbsp of thousand island onto the bun, followed by 4 or 5 dill pickle slices. **(B)** Next comes the sliced tomato, followed by a good amount of iceberg lettuce. Remember... this is a messy burger. **(C)** Place a cheeseburger patty on top of the lettuce, then a healthy scoop of the caramelized onions. **(D)** Lastly, spread 1 Tablespoon of dressing on the top bun. Done.

5. In case you're wondering why the recipe makes 4 burgers, but you only see 3 patties in these pictures... That's not a mistake. One was sacrificed as my wife's dinner. 👽😊

NOTES & SUGGESTIONS:

- *CHEESE:* Use any brand of "LOW POINT" sliced cheese you want. I used Velveeta Originals, because they are 1 point for 1 slice, 3 points for 2 and most people have access to them. Use whatever low point brand you can find and adjust your points. If you can find Borden Fat Free Cheddar Slices, those are 4 slices for 3 points.
- *DOUBLE DOUBLE ANIMAL:* Ok, you need to make this. The fabled In-n-Out Double Double Animal. It's the exact same process as this cheeseburger, but you're making a double cheeseburger. Add 1 more patty with cheese on top of the first patty, then place the onions on top. Look for pics on google for reference, if needed... and adjust your points.
- *ANIMAL STYLE:* Animal Style is an off-menu request, to have mustard fried onto the patties, along with caramelized onions and dressing on the top bun. A regular In-N-Out burger has none of that, it's a plain cheeseburger with a raw onion slice on top of the tomato, no mustard on the patties, no caramelized onions and no extra dressing. Ya'might as well order sadness.

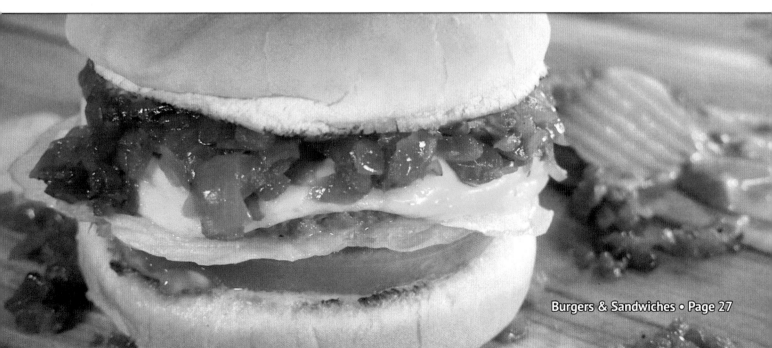

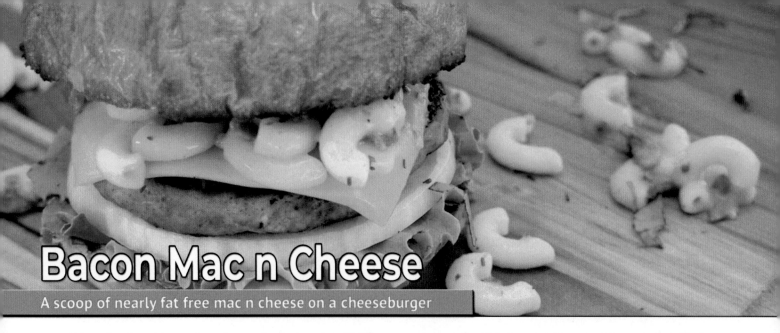

Bacon Mac n Cheese

A scoop of nearly fat free mac n cheese on a cheeseburger

When I set out to make a low calorie, low fat, FAST mac n cheese for this burger, I wanted to go a totally different route than most other recipes. I wanted to get the same texture and creaminess as old-school Kraft mac n cheese, where it's like the cheese powder packets. I didn't want it to require a bunch of melted cheese in heavy cream or half n half, so I had to get a little, dare I say.... Krafty? Seriously people... the cheese sauce only has 4g fat!

Servings Info.:

Yields: 4 burgers
Servings: 4
Serving Size: 1 burger

Points:

	G	B	P
1 serving =	4	4	2*
2 servings =	9	7	4*
3 servings =	13	11	5*
4 servings =	17	14	7*

(These listed points DO NOT INCLUDE the bun. Use whichever brand buns or bread you want, then add these points. This is what's between the buns. Purple points assume you are using 0 point macaroni.)

Ingredients:

Ground Turkey Patties:
- 1/2 batch of my 'Savory' ground turkey recipe, in my "Cookbook: Volume 1", on page 26. Form into 4 patties.

Quick Mac n Cheese: *(yields 1-1/3 cup)*
- 2 slices turkey bacon, cooked till crisp (see notes)***
- 3/4 cup chicken broth
- 2 slices fat free american or cheddar cheese slices. I used Borden's Fat Free Cheddar Slices. *(see notes)****
- 1/4 tsp salt
- 1/8 tsp turmeric (for color)
- 2 tsp cheese flavored popcorn seasoning *(optional)*
- 1 Tbsp cornstarch, dissolved in 1 Tbsp water, set aside.
- 1-1/3 cups cooked elbow macaroni noodles. If you're on the purple plan, use 0 point pasta, like whole wheat. (see notes)

Additional Ingredients:
- 4 slices of low point American or cheddar cheese. I used Borden's fat free cheddar slices for my recipe, but you can use any variety, such as Velveeta originals or Great Value brand.
- Lettuce or any preferred green leafy vegetable. I prefer 'green leafy' lettuce, it looks best in pictures.
- Sliced onion, white or red, your preference.
- Fresh Chives, finely chopped. (optional, for the mac.)

Directions:

1 Mix the meat and let it rest for 20 minutes. Form into 4 patties, set aside.

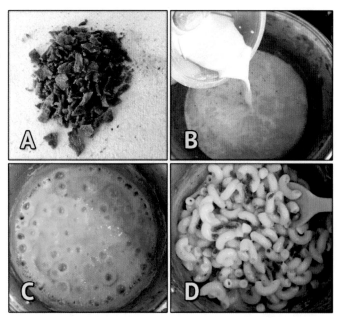

2 **(A)** Use cooking spray to cook bacon until crispy. Set aside so it hardens and cools. Chop into small bits. **(B)** In a small pot, bring the broth, cheese slices, salt, turmeric and popcorn seasoning (if using) to a low boil, stirring to melt the cheese. Once that is done, stir in the dissolved cornstarch. **(C)** Bring to a boil over medium heat and stir for 5 minutes. Turn off the heat and **(D)** stir in the cooked macaroni pasta and crispy bacon pieces. Mix to combine, then cover with lid and set aside. It will thicken more as it cools.

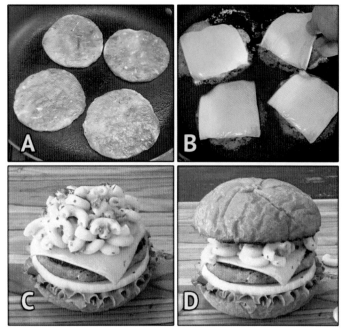

3 **(A)** Heat a large pan over medium heat for 1 minute. Spray with cooking spray, then cook the patties for 2 minutes. Flip the patties, **(B)** add the cheese slices, then cook for 2 more minutes. **(C)** To assemble the burgers, Toast your buns, then place some lettuce, then an onion slice onto the bun. Follow that with a burger patty, then place a 1/3 cup scoop of mac n cheese onto the patty. Sprinkle with chopped chives. **(D)** Scoop some bread out of the top bun, creating a crater, so that it will sit evenly on the mac n cheese. Place the bun on top of the mac, then press down gently. Done.

NOTES & SUGGESTIONS:

- *BACON NATION:* In this recipe, I used 2 points worth of turkey bacon. With the brand that I purchased, that gave me 2 slices. Feel free to use WHATEVER kind of bacon you want. Some brands give you more, some give you less. Want center cut pork bacon? Use it. Want Trader Joe's uncured turkey bacon? Awesome! You'll get 4 slices for 1 point! Use what you want, adjust points accordingly.
- *SLICED CHEESE:* I used Borden's Fat Free cheddar cheese slices. They are the lowest point and calorie, melty cheddar or American cheese I've found. However, not every store has them. In this recipe, all 6 slices of cheese, using Borden's FF cheese, are 4 points. In comparison, 6 slices of Velveeta Original slices are 9 points. Using Velveeta instead of the Borden's, raises the points of these burgers by 1 point per burger. If you use any cheese other than the Borden's, adjust your points.
- *CHEESE FLAVORED POPCORN SEASONING:* It's completely an optional ingredient. This sauce is plenty cheesy, but if you'd like an extra punch of cheese flavor, you can add in 2 teaspoons of most all brands of flavored cheese sprinkles. You can find them next to the popcorn in your grocery store. You can also use 'Molly McButter' brand, cheese sprinkles.
- *ELBOW MACARONI:* You Purple plan folks have no idea how jealous I am of you and your 0 point pasta. lol For this recipe, if you're on the purple plan and would like to use 'normal' pasta, use the points listed for the Blue plan. If however, you would like to use 0 point pasta, IE: whole wheat, garbanzo, black bean, whatever... pasta, I calculated the listed Purple points for that. If you DO use your 0 point pasta, feel free to add more cheese into the sauce. Mmmmmmmmmmmmm.... cheeeeese.

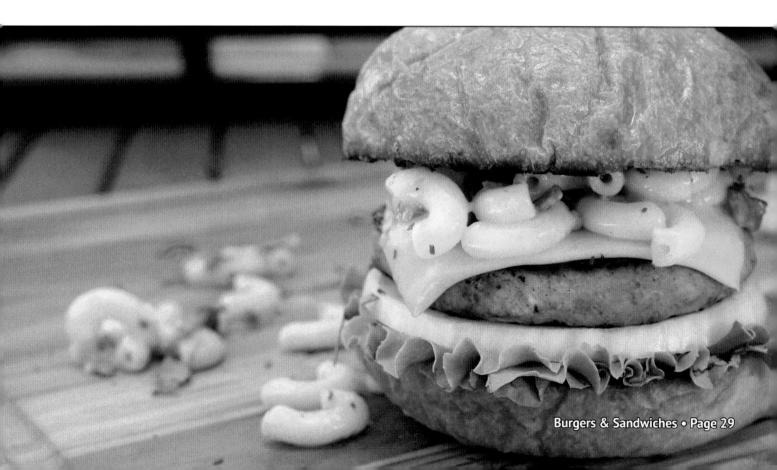

Bahn Mi Burger

A Vietnamese Classic, WW-ified into a Burger

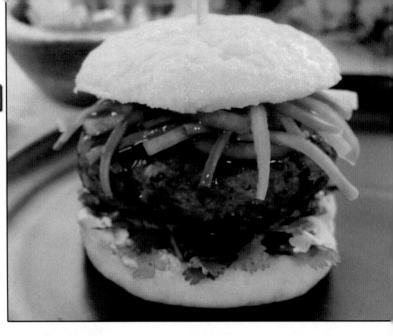

A Bahn Mi sandwich is a flavor and textural thing of beauty. In this case, you have a soft, steamed bun, with both a spicy and a savory sauce. Then you get the acidic crunch of pickled veggies, sliced cucumbers and aromatic herbs, on top of an aggressively seasoned chicken patty. This baby is bursting with asian flavors... it's like taking a trip to Danang, without having to get out of your pajamas.

Servings Info.:
Yields: 4 burgers
Servings: 4
Serving Size: 1 burger

Points:

	G	B	P
1 serving =	5	4	4
2 servings =	10	8	8
3 servings =	15	12	12
4 servings =	20	16	16

Ingredients:

EASY Pickled Vegetables
- 1 medium red onion, quartered and sliced thin
- 1 cup thin sliced carrots (bagged, shredded carrots work)
- 1 cup thin sliced, peeled, daikon radish or jicama, cut into thin strips, similar in size to the carrots you use.
- 3-4 jalapeno peppers, sliced into thin rounds. Remove seeds and the centers, if you want to cut down the spiciness.
- Distilled white vinegar and water, I used a 32oz bottle.

Steamed Asian-Style Buns
- 1 cup self rising flour
- 3/4 cup fat free greek yogurt
- 1 tsp baking powder
- additional water, as required, to juuuust form a dough ball.

Asian Ground Chicken Patties
- 1/2 batch of my "Asian" seasoned ground meat recipe, using ground CHICKEN BREAST instead of turkey. The recipe can be found in my "Cookbook: Volume 1", on page. 26.

Sriricha Yogurt Sauce
- 1/2 cup fat free Greek yogurt
- 1 Tbsp Sriracha chili sauce (to taste).
- 1 tsp reduced sodium soy sauce
- 1 tsp paprika (optional, for color)
- 1 tsp lime juice

Asian Dipping Sauce
- 1/4 cup of my sauce. The recipe can be found in my "Cookbook: Volume 1", on page 56.

Additional Vegetables
- 2 bunches fresh cilantro, rough chopped
- 1 cucumber, cut into thin slices, about as thick as a quarter.
- 2 Tbsp fresh mint, rough chopped

Directions:

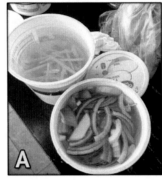
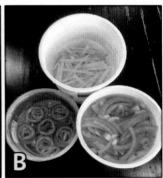

1. First things first... this is the easiest part. The night before you plan to make this, cut all of your veggies to be pickled. Place the sliced carrots and daikon radish (or jicama) in 1 container, the red onion in another, then the sliced and cleaned jalapenos in another. Use an equal amount of distilled white vinegar and water, to cover all of the veggies. Cover and set in the fridge overnight. Done.

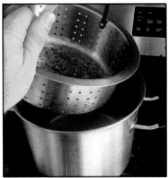
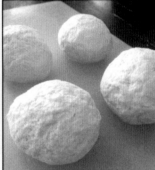

2. Fill a large pot, with a steamer insert basket, with 3-4" of water. Bring to a low boil, covered.

3. When you're ready to make the buns, combine the flour, yogurt and baking powder to form a dough ball. Use additional water if necessary. You want the dough to JUST come together. Section the ball into 1/4 cup balls.

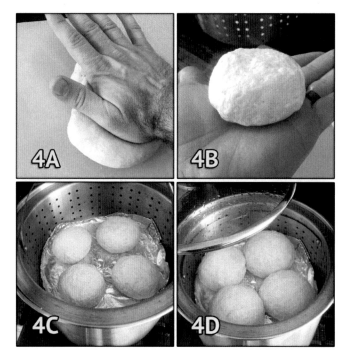

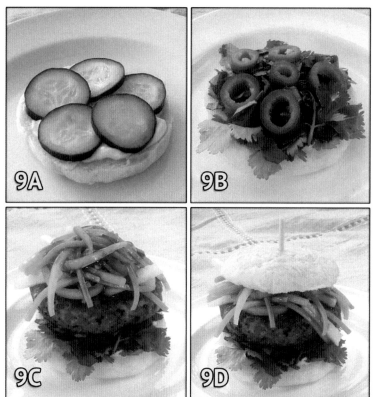

4. **(A)** Spray a cutting board with cooking spray, then use your palm to press one of the dough balls down. Fold it back over and onto itself, then press down again. Repeat 20 times then **(B)** roll into a smooth ball. **(C)** Place foil paper onto the bottom of your steamer insert, then place the rolled balls onto the foil. Place the insert into your pot, then cover, crank up the heat to medium-high, **(D)** then steam for 20 minutes.

5. Form the seasoned ground chicken into 4 patties. Cook in a frying pan with cooking spray. Set aside.

6. Take your steamed, cooled buns, then use a serrated knife to slice them horizontally, through the center.

7. Combine the ingredients for the Sriracha yogurt sauce and set aside in a dish, along with my asian dipping sauce, in a separate dish.

8. Get a buuuuunch of paper towels ready, or, you could use a few strainers, but I'm lazy, and hungry, so... Remove the various vegetables from their respective vinegar solutions. Place each bunch o' veggies, onto some paper towels and pat dry. You don't want a ton of vinegar dripping all over your burgers.

9. To assemble the burgers, first... **(A)** smear a dollop of the Sriracha yogurt on the bottom bun, followed by a few slices of cucumber. **(B)** Next, mix the chopped cilantro and mint together in a bowl, then place some of the fresh herbs on top of the cucumbers, followed by jalapeño rings, to taste. **(C)** Place a cooked chicken patty on top of the jalapeños, and top with a decent amount of the pickled vegetables. Drizzle 1 Tbsp of the Asian dipping sauce on top of the veggies.
(D) Finally, finish with the top bun and a skewer to hold it all in place. Done.

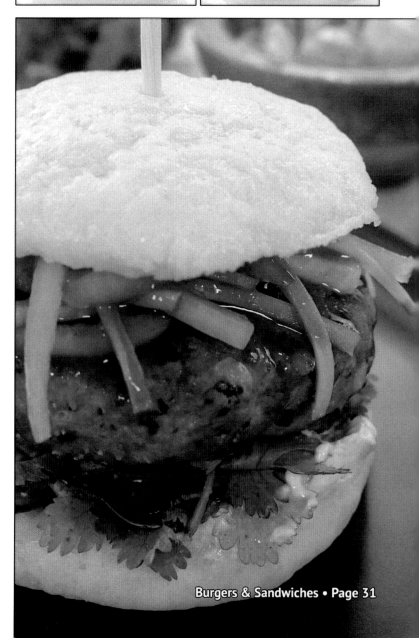

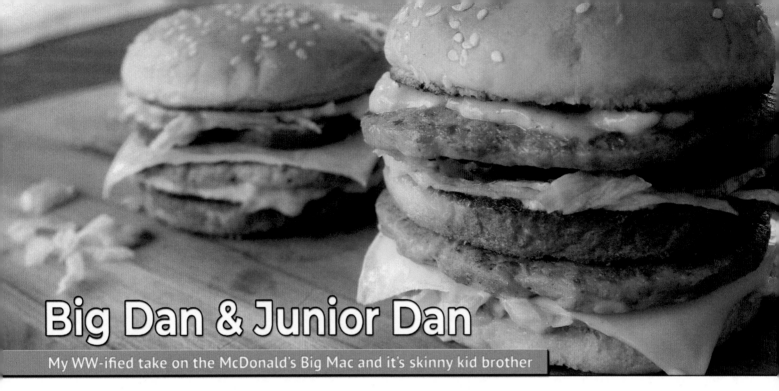

Big Dan & Junior Dan

My WW-ified take on the McDonald's Big Mac and it's skinny kid brother

This is my low point, low fat recipe for a McDonald's Big Mac, using ground turkey and my low point Thousand Island dressing. I'll also be showing you how to make a single patty version. Let's call them, **Big Dan** and **Junior Dan**. Best part? A REGULAR Big Mac is 18 points on all 3 plans, while mine has less points than a Laker game.

Now... sit down and put your thinking caps on, because this recipe is going to have a LOT of notes and WW-math.

Servings Info.:

Yields: 4 burgers
Servings: 4
Serving Size: 1 burger

Points:

	G	B	P
1 serving =	5(3)	3(2)	3(2)
2 servings =	10(6)	6(4)	6(4)
3 servings =	15(9)	8(5)	8(5)
4 servings =	20(12)	11(7)	11(7)

(These listed points DO NOT INCLUDE the top and bottom buns. The points on the left side of each column are for the "Double Patty" version. The lower points, in parentheses, are the point values for the single patty version. It's significantly lower on Green, because if you make the single patty version, you only need to make a 1/2 pound of ground turkey, as well as not needing the middle bun. The points also are factored as if you were using Velveeta Original cheese.)

Ingredients:

Savory Ground Turkey Patties:
- 1lb batch of my Savory Ground Turkey, recipe in my "Cookbook: Volume 1", on page 30, formed into (8) 2oz patties.

Low Point Thousand Island Dressing:
- 1 batch of my Thousand Island dressing, recipe on page 21.

Additional Ingredients:
- 4 slices of low point american cheese slices, such as Borden's Fat Free singles (3 points), or Velveeta Original (6 points)***
- 1/2 head of Iceberg lettuce, finely shredded.
- 1 medium white onion, finely diced
- Dill pickle slices, at least 4 per burger.
- An entire package of 8 burger buns (see notes)***

Directions:

The following instructions are the process to make the double decker "Big Dan" burger. Instructions will also be provided for making the single patty version.

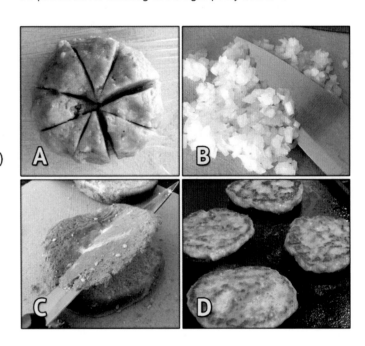

1. **(A)** Roll your 1 lb of ground turkey into a mound, then use a knife to cut it into 8 equal sections. Shape the meat into patties, set aside to rest for 20 minutes. **(B)** Finely dice the onion, set aside.. **(C)** Take the bottom bun from each of the extra 4 hamburger buns in the package, then use a knife to slice off a the dark, baked bottom. You want to have white bread on both sides. By weight, it should be 1 point of bread. **(D)** Preheat a pan over medium heat for 1 minute, then cook the burger patties for 2 minutes on each side. Done.

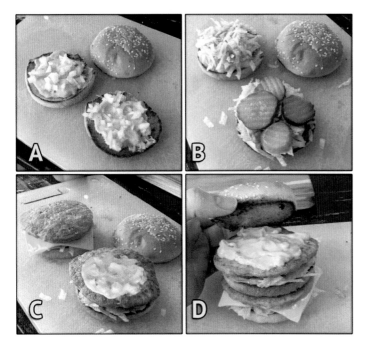

- *CHEESE:* There is a major variable in this recipe. It is the points for the cheese. I found a Fat Free brand of cheddar cheese slices in my grocery store's cheese section, it's the "Borden's" brand, fat free cheddar singles. They let you have up to 5 slices for 3 points. Velveeta Originals are also low point cheese slices. They are 6 points for 4 slices. I formulated this recipe with the higher point Velveeta slices, because they are easier for people to find. I'd highly suggest scanning your local store brands and adjust your points if needed.

- *MIDDLE BUN:* For these 4 burgers… we are going to need an extra "bottom bun", that we can slice and use as the middle piece of bread. Burger buns are sold in packs of 8. I took the remaining 4 burger buns and used the extra bottom 'round' from the extra 4 buns. As seen in picture "1C", I sliced the 'browned' bread off of the bottom of the 4 extra bottom buns. That allowed me to have the middle bun be 1 point, by weight. Weigh the bun, using your kitchen scale, in grams. You want it to be 1 point of bread. If you are using high point buns, figure out the points for your bread by weighing it, then adjust the points in this recipe. I used generic store brand, 4 point buns for mine.

2. To assemble 'The Big Dan', first toast the buns. **(A)** Place a dollop of thousand island onto both the bottom and the middle buns, followed by some diced onions. **(B)** Next, place some shredded lettuce onto both buns. On what will be the center bun, arrange a few pickle slices. **(C)** Place a slice of cheese on top of the lettuce, on the bottom bun (left bun), then a smear of dressing onto the top patty. **(D)** Stack it all together, with the top half onto the bottom half, then cover with top bun.

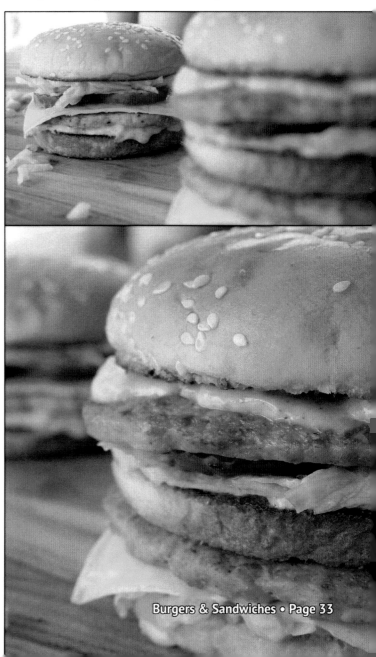

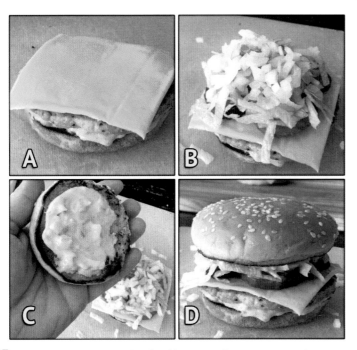

3. To assemble the 'Junior Dan' burgers, first, toast your buns.
(A) Smear the bottom bun with some thousand island, then place a burger patty on top, followed by 1 slice of cheese.
(B) Place pickles on top of the cheese, followed by a mound of shredded lettuce, then top the lettuce with diced onions.
(C) Smear some thousand island onto the top bun, **(D)** then cap the burger with the bun. Done.

Blue Cheese & Balsamic Onions

Caramelized balsamic onions with savory blue cheese funk

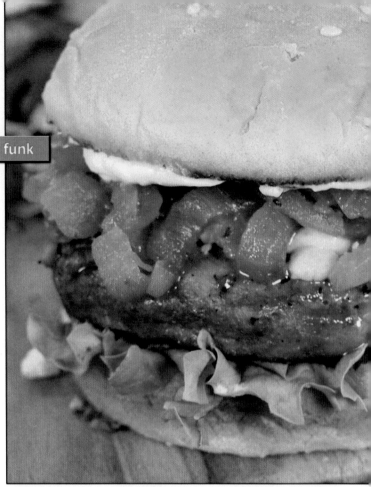

This is one of those swanky types of burgers, typically found on the menu at a sit down restaurant, rather than coming out of your kitchen. The strong flavor of blue cheese gets mellowed out by the caramelized balsamic onions, that lend a sweetness to the burger. Though I use a 1/4lb patty, you could use a smaller 2oz patty to save points on Green.

Servings Info.:
Yields: 4 burgers
Servings: 4
Serving Size: 1 burger

Points:

	G	B	P
1 serving =	4	2	2
2 servings =	8	3	3
3 servings =	11	5	5
4 servings =	15	6	6

*(These listed points **DO NOT INCLUDE** the bun. Use whichever brand buns or bread you want, then add these points.)*

Ingredients:

Savory Ground Turkey Patties **
• 1lb batch of my Savory Ground Turkey, recipe in my "Cookbook: Volume 1", on page 30.

Garlic Aioli Spread
• 6 Tbsp fat free plain Greek yogurt
• 3-1/2 tsp light mayonnaise
• 1 tsp lemon juice
• 2 medium garlic cloves, crushed and minced
• 1/4 tsp garlic powder
• pinch of salt and pepper

Caramelized Balsamic Onions:
• 2 large yellow onions sliced into strips
• 1 medium garlic clove crushed and minced
• 4 second spray, butter flavored cooking spray (0 point)
• 2 tsp onion powder
• 1/4 tsp salt
• 1/4 tsp black pepper
• 1/2 cup fat free beef broth
• 1 Tbsp white vinegar
• 2 tsp balsamic vinegar

Additional Ingredients:
• 4 Tbsp PLUS 2 tsp Blue Cheese
• Lettuce, any preferred variety

Directions:

1. Mix all of the Aioli ingredients together in a cup, or other sealable container. Set aside for at least 30 minutes, for the flavors to meld.

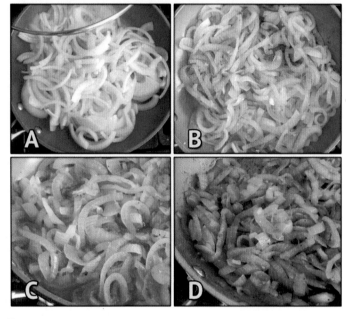

2. (A) Place the onions and garlic in a large pan over medium heat. Spray with a 4 second spray of butter flavored cooking spray, cover with a lid, **(B)** then cook for 10 minutes, stirring occasionally to ensure they don't burn. **(C)** After 10 minutes, stir in the onion powder, salt, pepper, beef broth, white vinegar and balsamic vinegar. **(D)** Cook, uncovered, for 8-10 more minutes, until all of the excess liquid has evaporated. Set aside. This can be made up to 2 days in advance and stored in the fridge. Reheat prior to serving.

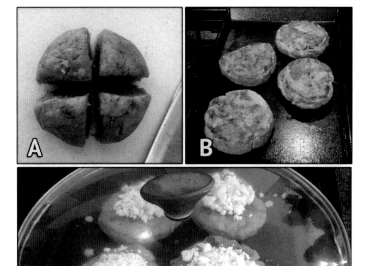

- *CHEESE:* Though this IS a blue cheese burger, the blue cheese is relatively mild. If you want to use more, you can add an additional 4 Tablespoons of blue cheese, which would let you have 1 more Tablespoon on top of each burger... and the burgers would only go up by 1 point per serving. Heck, if you want to use reduced fat blue cheese, feel free. I couldn't because no stores around me have it.
- Don't like Blue Cheese? You can also use Gorgonzola.
- These are THICK 1/4lb patty burgers, which are 2 points each on the GREEN plan. If you GREEN folks want to save a point, use a thinner 2oz patty, like on my other burgers.
- The onions and aioli can be made ahead of time.

3. **(A)** Take your pre-mixed 1lb batch of my savory ground turkey and section it into 4 equal 1/4's. **(B)** Form the 1/4 pound sections into patties and cook with cooking spray. **(C)** When the burgers are almost finished, cover each patty with 1 Tbsp PLUS 1/2 tsp of crumbled blue cheese, pour a little water in the pan and immediately cover with a lid, to melt the cheese.

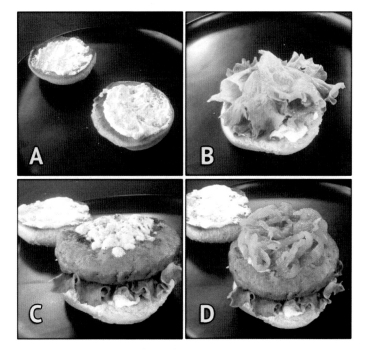

4. To assemble the burgers, first toast the buns, then **(A)** smear a scoop of the garlic aioli onto both buns. **(B)** Place a layer of lettuce over the spread, **(C)** followed by one of the blue cheese-topped burger patties. **(D)** Place a good sized serving of the caramelized onions on top of the blue cheese, then cover with the top bun. Done.

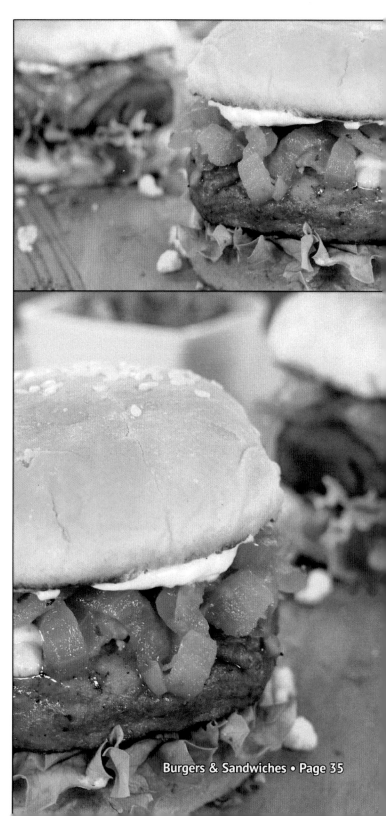

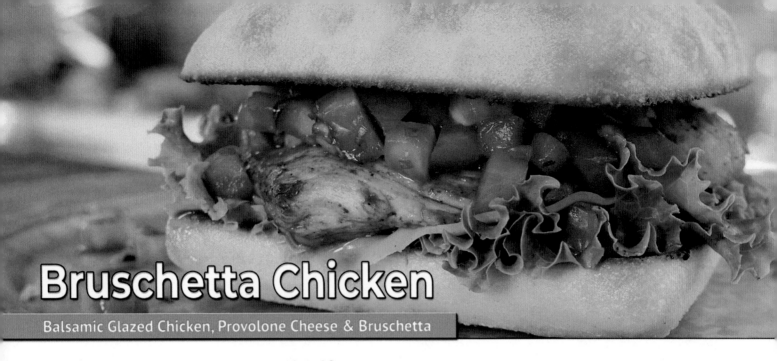

Bruschetta Chicken

Balsamic Glazed Chicken, Provolone Cheese & Bruschetta

This simple sandwich is light, fresh and full of flavor. We simply season chicken breasts with salt and pepper, then glaze it with a sweet and tangy balsamic syrup. It then gets served with provolone cheese, lettuce, and a big scoop of bruschetta, then drizzled with the balsamic pan sauce.

Ingredients:

Chicken Breasts:
- (4) 4oz boneless, skinless chicken breasts.

Simple Bruschetta:
- 1-1/4 large tomato, diced (around 1 cup).
- 1/4 cup fresh basil, loosely packed, finely chopped.
- 2 medium garlic cloves, finely chopped
- 1/2 tsp salt
- 1/4 tsp pepper
- 1/4 tsp olive oil
- 1-1/2 tsp balsamic vinegar
-

Balsamic Glaze:
- 2 Tbsp balsamic vinegar
- 2 Tbsp red wine vinegar
- 1 Tbsp sugar free pancake syrup

Additional Ingredients:
- 4 slices thin sliced provolone cheese (see notes)
- Lettuce, whichever variety you prefer. I used 'Green Leaf' lettuce. It looks nicest in pictures, in my opinion.

Directions:

1. Mix together all of the ingredients for the bruschetta. Place in a bowl, cover with plastic wrap and set in the fridge for at least an hour.

2. In a small bowl, stir together the balsamic glaze ingredients. Set aside.

Servings Info.:	Points:	G	B	P
Yields: 4 sandwiches	1 serving =	4	2	2
Servings: 4	2 servings =	8	4	4
Serving Size: 1 sandwich	3 servings =	11	6	6
	4 servings =	15	8	8

(These listed points DO NOT INCLUDE the bun. Use whichever brand buns or bread you want, then add these points. This is what's between the buns)

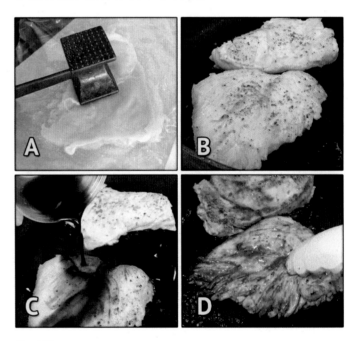

3. **(A)** Lightly pound the chicken breasts to make them cook more evenly, they'll also shrink less. **(B)** Heat a pan for 1 minute over medium heat. Season chicken with salt and pepper, spray with cooking spray on both sides, then add to the pan. Cook over medium heat for 2 minutes, flip, then cook for 2 additional minutes. **(C)** Pour the balsamic glaze into the pan with the chicken. Allow the chicken to cook for 1 minute, moving it around the pan. **(D)** Flip the chicken and cook for 1 more minute, coating with the thickened sauce. Set aside.

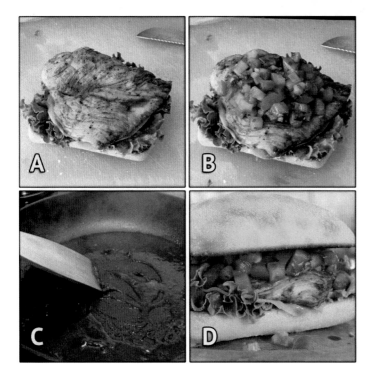

4. **(A)** Toast your bread o' choice, then place some lettuce onto the bottom bun, followed by a slice of the provolone cheese. Set one of the glazed chicken breasts on top of the cheese, then get your bruschetta out of the fridge. **(B)** Place a 1/4 cup scoop of bruschetta on top of the chicken, arranging it into a nice mound. **(C)** Now, heat up the pan you used to cook the chicken in. Pour in a little water, to deglaze the pan and create a little more thickened balsamic sauce. Drizzle some of the sauce onto the bruschetta of each sandwich. **(D)** Cover with the top bun.

NOTES & SUGGESTIONS:

- *BRUSCHETTA:* I always joke that Bruschetta is just the Italian version of Pico de Gallo. This is a simple, no frills Bruschetta recipe. You can bulk it up if you'd like, by adding some diced onion, or more tomato.
- *BALSAMIC GLAZE:* This is my low point take on a Honey Balsamic pan sauce. Rather than using honey, I'm using sugar free pancake syrup. Feel free to use regular maple syrup, or even to use honey... but adjust your points.
- *CHEESE:* 1 slice of thin sliced sargento brand provolone is 1 point and 40 calories. NORMAL sliced provolone is usually 3 to 4 points per slice. If you can't find thin sliced provolone cheese at your supermarket, go to the deli section and ask them to slice some provolone for you. Yes... ask them to cut the cheese. Finish chuckling like a potty mouthed 8 year old, then tell them you want **VERY** thin slices, not regular thickness. When you get home, weigh a slice with your kitchen scale, so that you can see how many points your freshly sliced cheese is, by weight in grams. MOST grocery stores sell thin or ultra thin sliced provolone though. If you can't find ultra thin sliced provolone, or your store's deli department can't thin slice it for you, feel free to use thin sliced mozzarella. Any packaged cheese that is 40 calories or less for the first slice is usually 1 point for the first slice, 3 points for two slices.

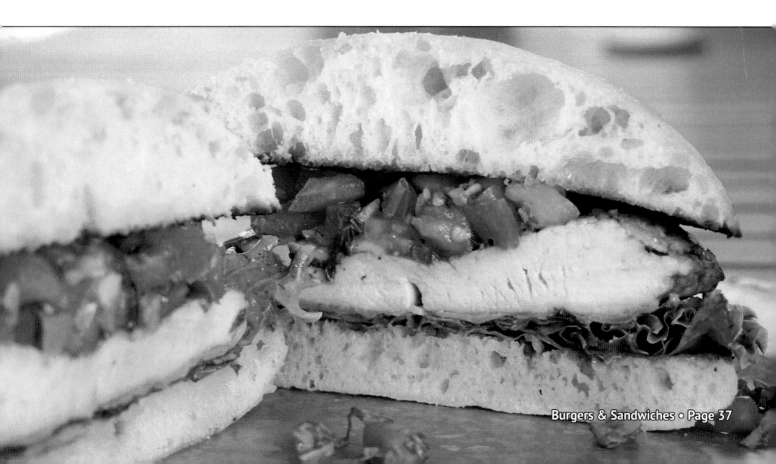

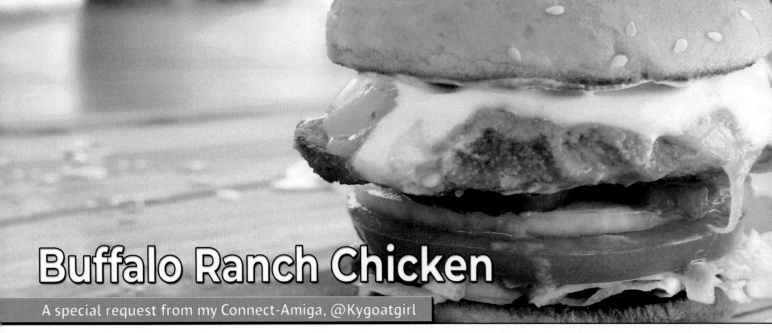

Buffalo Ranch Chicken

A special request from my Connect-Amiga, @Kygoatgirl

This is my WW-ified version of the sandwich from the national food chain, "Buffalo Wild WIngs". My version uses a chicken breast that's been breaded and baked with my low point breading recipe. It then gets topped with Swiss cheese and drizzled with low point ranch dressing and buffalo sauce.

Ingredients:

Breaded Chicken Breasts:
• 4 chicken breasts. For you Greenies, use 4oz chicken breasts.
• Breading: Prepare 1 batch of my "breading 2.0", recipe in my "Cookbook: Volume 1", on page 35. However, if you're on the Green Plan, use egg whites instead of whole eggs, for points.

Quick Buffalo Sauce: (makes 1 cup, 0 total points)
• 3/4 cup 0 point red pepper sauce, such as 'Frank's RedHot original cayenne pepper sauce'.
• 2 tsp worcestershire sauce
• 2 Tbsp white vinegar
• 1/2 tsp garlic powder
• 2 Tbsp plain fat free Greek yogurt

Quick Ranch Dressing:
• 3/4 cup plain fat free Greek yogurt
• 1/4 cup almond milk, or water
• 1 tsp light mayonnaise
• 1-2 tsp Hidden Valley 'Ranch' dressing & seasoning mix. Buy a ranch dressing packet from the store. Scan it to ensure you get one that's 0 points for at least half of the packet.

Additional Ingredients:
• 4 slices thin sliced Swiss cheese (see notes)
• Dill pickle slices
• Sliced Onion
• 4 tomato slices
• Lettuce

Servings Info.:	Points:	G	B	P
Yields: 4 sandwiches	1 serving =	5	3	3
Servings: 4	2 servings =	10	5	5
Serving Size: 1 sandwich	3 servings =	14	8	8
	4 servings =	19	10	10

(These listed points DO NOT INCLUDE the bun. Use whichever brand buns or bread you want, then add these points. This is what's between the buns)

Directions:

1. Prepare a batch of my breading, as directed. Set aside. Mix together the Buffalo sauce. Set aside. Mix together the ranch dressing. Set aside.

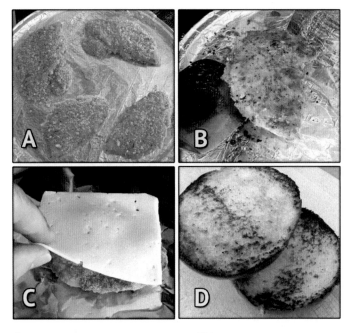

2. Preheat oven to 425 degrees. **(A)** Bread the chicken, spray with cooking spray and bake for 14 minutes. **(B)** Flip and cook for 8 more minutes. **(C)** Remove from oven, place 1 slice of cheese onto each breast (the chicken ones!!!) Bake for 1 more minute, to melt the cheese. **(D)** Toast the buns, set aside.

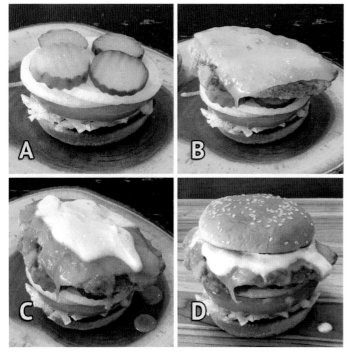

3. **(A)** Place a small mound of lettuce onto your bottom bun, followed by a slice of tomato, then onion rounds and dill pickle slices. **(B)** Next, place a cheese covered chicken breast on top of the pickles. **(C)** Pour a scoop of buffalo sauce on top of the cheese, then drizzle a good amount of ranch dressing onto the buffalo sauce. **(D)** Finally, place the toasted top bun onto the sandwich. Go grab a fist full of napkins, unhinge your jaw, and get to work. Done.

NOTES & SUGGESTIONS:

- **CHICKEN:** If you choose to simply grill or cook the chicken in a pan, without breading it, your sandwiches will go down 1 point per sandwich.
- **BUFFALO SAUCE:** This is a simple, quick, easy and slightly creamy buffalo sauce. However, it is a thinner sauce, because it's meant to be drizzled and not to be used as a thick dip. If you would LIKE the sauce to be thicker, there are 2 options:
  * Mix in some more Greek yogurt. This will make it thicker, but will cut back on the spiciness. However, it will add points for Greenies.
  * In a small pot, bring the first 4 ingredients to a boil. Pour in 1-1/2 tsp cornstarch, dissolved into 1 Tbsp of water. Let it boil for 1-2 minutes, then allow to cool. Once cooled, stir in the Greek yogurt.
- **RANCH:** You don't have to make mine, use whatever Ranch you want, but adjust your points.
- **BREADING:** You Gluten Free folks, please make note that KELLOGG'S brand Rice Krispies is not Gluten free. Make sure to find a gluten free brand, or use another cereal that is low points for 1-1/4 cups, such as rice chex.
- **CHEESE:** 2 slices of Sargento brand thin sliced swiss cheese are 3 points. NORMAL thickness swiss cheese is usually 3 points. So, it gives you options. You can use 1 thin slice per sandwich, like I did, which makes the points for the cheese 1 point on the first burger, 3 for the second, 4 for the 3rd and 6 for the 4th serving of cheese. Or, you can simply scan different brands of Swiss cheese, use whatever you want, and adjust the points of the recipe. Either way... it's a low point sandwich.
- **SPICINESS:** Want the sandwich spicier? After the chicken first comes out of the oven, dunk the breasts in buffalo sauce, then place back on the pan, cover with cheese, THEN put back into the oven to melt the cheese.

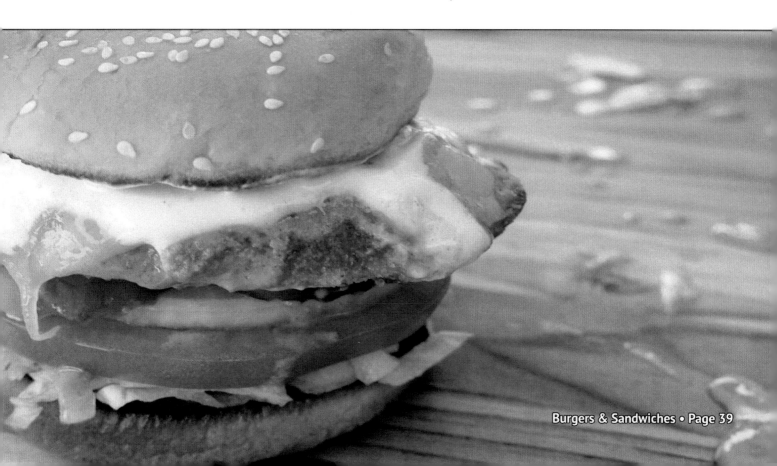

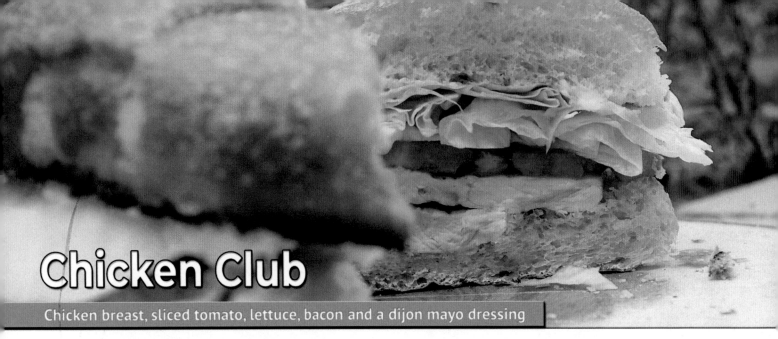

Chicken Club

Chicken breast, sliced tomato, lettuce, bacon and a dijon mayo dressing

I was making my wife a sandwich for dinner, but all there was in the fridge was a tomato, some leftover lettuce and 2 pieces of turkey bacon. We've all been there. You open the fridge and feel like you're on an episode of 'Chopped'. So... an easy, tasty, no fuss BLT with chicken, seemed to be the right call. I decided to use a dijon mayonnaise spread, rather than just plain mayo, to kick the sandwich up a bit, because 'simple' doesn't mean you can't have a little 'tude.

Servings Info.:
Yields: 4 sandwiches
Servings: 4
Serving Size: 1 sandwich

Points:

	G	B	P
1 serving =	4	2	2
2 servings =	8	4	4
3 servings =	11	5	5
4 servings =	15	7	7

(These listed points DO NOT INCLUDE the bun. Use whichever brand buns or bread you want, then add these points. This is what's between the buns)

Ingredients:

Chicken Breasts:
• Ok, here's the deal. You can use (4) 4oz chicken breasts, OR you can use (8) 2oz chicken breast tenderloins. Ideally, you want to use the larger breasts... but because of grocery ridiculousness during COVID, I had to make this sandwich with 2 tenderloins (pictured). It's what I had on hand.

Dijon/Mayo spread:
• 1/2 cup plain fat free Greek yogurt
• 1 tsp light mayonnaise
• 2 tsp dijon mustard
• 1/8 tsp salt

Additional Toppings:
• 8 slices low point turkey bacon. Use whatever type of bacon you want, but if you go over 2 points per sandwich, adjust the points for this recipe.
• 4 tomato slices
• Any lettuce or green-leafy-variety-type-thingie o' choice, I used Iceberg lettuce.

Directions:

1. Mix all of the dijon mayo ingredients together till well combined. Set aside.

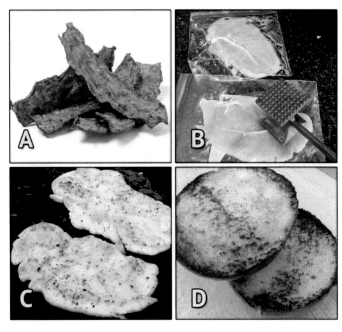

2. **(A)** Spray the turkey bacon with cooking spray, then fry in a pan until crispy. Set aside. **(B)** Place your chicken into plastic bags and use a kitchen mallet, small pot, or a receipt from CVS Pharmacy to thin them out a bit. Don't kill them, just give 'em a few love taps. **(C)** Season with salt and pepper, preheat the same pan for 1 minute over medium heat, then add the chicken. Cook for 1-1/2 minutes per side (for thin tenderloins). Set aside. **(D)** Toast your buns (the burger buns, <u>not yours</u>) and set aside.

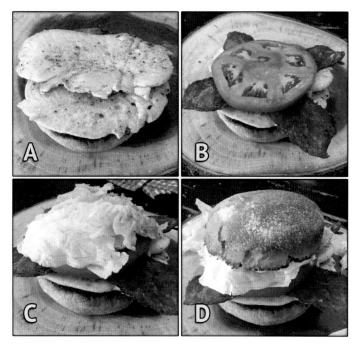

A B

C D

3. **(A)** Place the 2 chicken tenderloins onto your bottom bun.
(B) Cross 2 pieces of bacon over the chicken, then top with a slice of tomato. **(C)** Place a mound of lettuce on top of the tomato, then go get your dijon mayo out of the fridge. **(D)**. Smear 2 Tablespoons of the dijon mayo spread onto the top bun, then set it onto the lettuce. Done.

NOTES & SUGGESTIONS:

- *CHICKEN:* I would preferred to use a 4oz chicken breast for this sandwich. However, all that I had was small tenderloins in my freezer... so... you use what'cha have. If you use chicken breasts, you'll obviously need to increase the cooking time by a few minutes per side.
- *DAIRY FREE MAYO SPREAD:* Want to make this, but you're allergic to dairy and can't have the mayo or yogurt? No problem. A low point fix is as easy as simply blending 1/2 cup of semi-firm (medium) tofu with 2-3 Tbsp of water. Add a little splash of lemon juice to help give it some tang. Is it exaaaactly like mayo and yogurt? No. But, it's a good low point substitute for folks with allergies.
- *BACON:* I calculated the points for this recipe with 2 points of bacon per sandwich. If you are able to purchase a specific brand that give you more bacon for 2 points, I'm looking at YOU, Trader Joe's... use what you want. Just make sure to adjust your points if you end up using more than 2 points of bacon per sandwich. If you end up using a brand that gives you 2 pieces for LESS than 1 point each.... you can reduce the points per sandwich. Meaning: If you use a brand of bacon that lets you have 2 slices for 1 point... then each of your sandwiches costs 1 less point than what I have listed.
- *VANISHING BACON?:* You may be wondering why the nice picture on the left page doesn't have any bacon in it. Well, that pic happened by accident. I made the sandwich, took the picture below (with bacon), then had to remove the bacon for my wife... she doesn't like it on sandwiches. When she sliced it open, to eat it, she said "hey, this'd be a nice picture!" Of course, she said that right as I had stuffed her 2 unwanted pieces of bacon into my mouth. So... no bacon in that pic. Use your imagination.

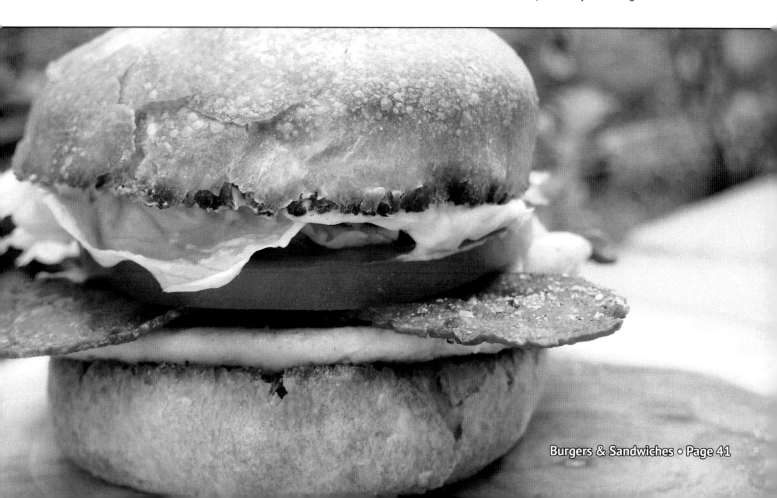

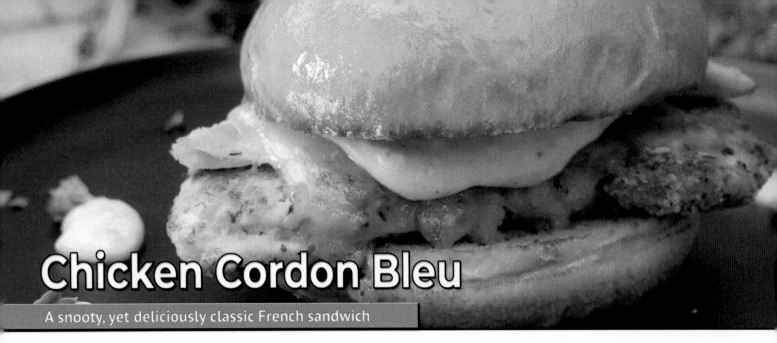

Chicken Cordon Bleu

A snooty, yet deliciously classic French sandwich

I have to confess that I haven't had many of these sandwiches in my lifetime. I've never been a huge fan of honey mustard sauces... luckily, this isn't honey mustard, it's a maple mustard. I decided to go a little non-traditional to save on points. The flavor is just as good and cuts the heck out of the calories. In this version, we're using my low point "breading 2.0" recipe to coat and bake chicken breasts. They are then covered with 3 slices of deli ham, topped with light swiss cheese and tossed back in the oven to melt. Finally, the sandwich is finished off with a good dollop of maple mustard spread. Viva la France!

Ingredients:

Breaded Chicken Breasts:
- 4 chicken breasts. For you greenies, use chicken that's no more than 1 point per breast.
- Breading: Prepare 1 batch of my "breading 2.0", recipe in my "Cookbook: Volume 1", on page 35. However, do not add the dijon mustard to the egg wash.

Maple Mustard Dressing/Sauce:
- 2-1/2 Tbsp plain fat free Greek yogurt
- 1 Tbsp dijon mustard
- 1 Tbsp organic stone ground mustard (scan for a brand that gives you 1 Tbsp for 0 points)
- 2 Tbsp traditional yellow mustard
- 1 Tbsp sugar free maple syrup (pancake syrup)
- 1 tsp light mayonnaise
- 1/2 tsp 0 point sweetener o' choice
- 1/4 tsp black pepper
- 1 Tbsp lemon juice
- dash of hot sauce (optional, to taste)

Additional Toppings:
- 12 slices deli ham (or up to 4 points worth of ham)
- 4 slices of light, thin sliced, or reduced fat swiss cheese, such as Jarlsberg brand. (see notes)**

Directions:

1. Prepare a batch of my breading, as directed. Set aside.

2. Mix all of the maple mustard ingredients together till smooth, set aside.

Servings Info.:
Yields: 4 burgers
Servings: 4
Serving Size: 1 burger

Points:

	G	B	P
1 serving =	4	3	3
2 servings =	9	7	7
3 servings =	13	10	10
4 servings =	18	14	15

(These listed points DO NOT INCLUDE the bun. Use whichever brand buns or bread you want, then add these points. This is what's between the buns)

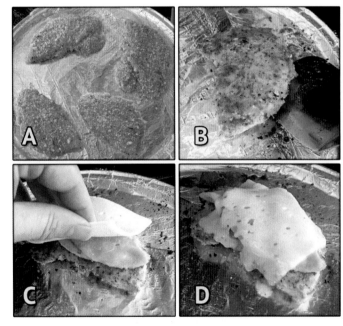

3. Preheat oven to 425 degrees. **(A)** Bread the chicken, spray with cooking spray and bake for 12 minutes. **(B)** Flip and cook for 8 more minutes. **(C)** Remove from oven, place 3 slices of ham onto the chicken, followed by a slice of the Swiss. **(D)** Bake for 1 more minute, to melt the cheese.

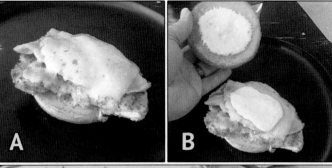

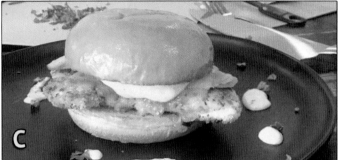

4. **(A)** Toast your sandwich buns o' choice, then place one of the breaded, baked chicken breasts on top. **(B)** Scoop one Tablespoon of mustard sauce on top of the melted Swiss cheese, then spread one additional Tablespoon of mustard sauce onto the top bun. You don't want to plop both scoops onto the chicken, otherwise it'll look like a can of pale yellow paint got dumped on your sandwich. **(C)** Forget to to clean off your kitchen counter before taking the last picture of your sandwich… just like me. Done.

NOTES & SUGGESTIONS:

- **CHICKEN:** Blue & Purple folks can use Dolly Parton sized chicken breasts, however, you Green folks should use chicken that is an appropriate size (in ounces) to not go go above 1 point per sandwich.
- **MAPLE MUSTARD?:** (whiny voice) "But… but… what about Honey Mustard?" Simple, Honey has more points than a Powerpoint lecture. Sugar free pancake (maple) syrup doesn't. It's common knowledge at this point that my recipes lean towards reduced sugar and sugar free in nature… because 1) Points, and 2) Diabetics. You can use a low point honey mustard dressing, like G. Hughes, if you'd like. If you do, adjust your points.
- **BREADING:** My Rice Krispies breading recipe is lower in points and calories than an equal amount of regular breading. However, you Gluten Free folks, please make note that KELLOGG'S brand Rice Krispies is not Gluten Free. Make sure to find a gluten free brand, or use another cereal that is low points for 1-1/4 cups, such as rice chex.
- **HAM:** Different brands of sliced deli ham have different calorie counts and points per serving. Scan the packages. You want to have around 4oz for 3-4 points, which should give you 12 slices. I used Oscar Mayer, deli fresh, uncured.
- **CHEESE:** 2 slices of Sargento brand thin sliced swiss cheese are 3 points. NORMAL thickness swiss cheese is usually 3 points. So, it gives you options. You can use 1 thin slice per sandwich, like I did, which makes the points for the cheese 1 point on the first burger, 3 for the second, 4 for the 3rd and 6 for the 4th serving of cheese. Or, you can simply scan different brands of Swiss cheese, use whatever you want, and adjust the points of the recipe. Either way… it's a low point sandwich.

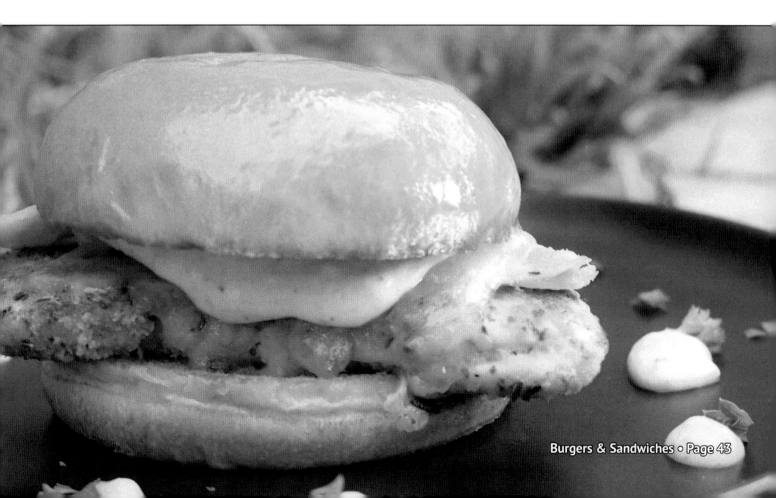

Chicken Parmesan

With provolone, marinara and roasted garlic spread

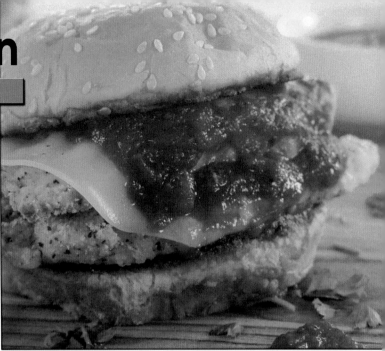

I love, love, love chicken parmesan sandwiches. Whenever my wife wasn't around and I wanted to gorge on a calorie heavy sandwich (back when I was still fat Dan), I'd order one from a local pizza place and eat it before she got home. THIS version is a delicious and muuuuch healthier version. We're lowering the points of the breading by using my crushed rice krispies breading, as well as thin sliced provolone cheese. In order to impart even MORE flavor, we're roasting cloves of garlic with cooking spray, rather than olive oil…then spreading it on each of the buns, turning them into awesome roasted garlic buns, for 0 additional points. Boomshakalaka.

Servings Info.:
Yields: 4 sandwiches
Servings: 4
Serving Size: 1 sandwich

Points:

	G	B	P
1 serving =	4	3*	3*
2 servings =	8	5	5
3 servings =	11	8	8
4 servings =	15	10	10

*(These listed points **DO NOT INCLUDE** the bun. Use whichever brand buns or bread you want, then add these points. These listed points are also for 5oz of chicken.)*

Ingredients:

Chicken: (see notes)
- 8 chicken breast tenderloins, 2 for each sandwich. When weighed, mine averaged 5oz for the 2.***

QUICK Marinara Sauce:
- 1 batch of my "5 minute marinara sauce", recipe on page 14.

Low Point Breading:
1 batch of my "Low Point Breading 2.0, from Cookbook 1,
- recipe on page 35, with the following changes:
  - If you are on the Green plan, use egg whites instead of whole eggs, to save points.
  - Add 2 tsp reduced fat kraft grated parmesan topping.

Additional Ingredients:
10 OR MORE medium garlic cloves, use as much as you want.
- 4 slices of "ulta thin" deli sliced provolone cheese, such as
- sargento or jarlsberg brand.*** (see notes)
  Fresh basil, optional
-

Directions:

1. Prepare 1 batch of 0 point marinara sauce, set aside.

2. Prepare a batch of my low point breading 2.0, with the listed changes. Set the dry ingredients in one shallow bowl and then beat the eggs (or egg whites) in another. Store the egg wash in the fridge, till ready.

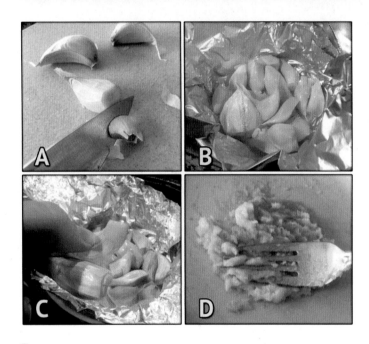

3. **(A)** Slice the ends off of at least 10 fresh garlic cloves, still in the skin. **(B)** Place all of the garlic into a pouch made of tin foil, then spray with cooking spray. Close the foil pouch and bake at 375 degrees for 45 minutes. **(C)** Remove from oven, then pick up each garlic clove and gently squeeze the back end, which will cause the roasted garlic to fall out. Place all garlic cloves into a dish. **(D)** Add 2 tsp water to the garlic cloves, then mash with a fork till smooth. Seal in an air tight container and set aside.

4. Take 2 chicken breast tenderloins, which should be around 5oz of skinless boneless chicken breast, and place them into a gallon sized ziplock bag. Use a kitchen mallet, rolling pin, or a small cooking pot to pound the chicken thin. You just want to flatten them a bit, you don't want to obliterate them. Continue until all of the chicken has been beaten and mugged. Set aside.

5. Heat your oven to 425 degrees and line a baking pan with foil, spray with cooking spray. Dip each thinned chicken breast piece into the egg wash, then lightly bread each side with the crumb mixture. LIGHTLY, there will JUST be enough to coat them all. Bake at 425 degrees for 20-22 minutes. Remove from oven.

6. To assemble the sandwiches, toast the buns, then **(A)** spread some of the mashed garlic onto each bun. **(B)** Place 2 chicken cutlets on top of each other, then **(C)** place a slice of provolone on the chicken, followed by a scoop of hot marinara sauce. **(D)** Finally, top the sandwich with the top bun. Done.

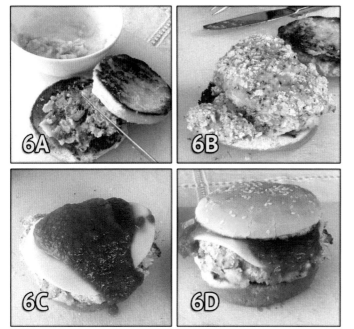

NOTES & SUGGESTIONS:

- *POINTS:* I used 2 thin chicken breast pieces, which both came to around 5 ounces. YOU can choose to use a single 5 ounce chicken breast, if you'd like. It will save you prep time and would require using less breading. It might even allow you to double coat each breast in crumbs, resulting in crispier baked chicken. It's totally up to you, whether you'd like to go with 2 small chicken breast strips that get pounded, or just use a single 5oz strip. People on Blue and Purple don't have to worry about it, but this is mainly for folks on GREEN, who count points for chicken breast.

  ALSO: Though it says the first serving is 3 points on Blue & Purple, that's with all of the ingredients across all 4 burgers, including all 4 slices (6 points) of cheese. Honestly, if you're only eating 1 of these, I'd personally count it as 2 points for the "filling" (on blue & purple), not 3 points. 1 point is for the chicken's breading and 1 point is for the single slice of cheese on your 1 single sandwich.

- *CHEESE:* 1 slice of thin sliced sargento brand provolone is 1 point and 40 calories. NORMAL sliced provolone is usually 3 to 4 points per slice. If you can't find thin sliced provolone cheese at your supermarket, go to the deli section and ask them to slice some provolone for you. Yes... ask them to cut the cheese. Finish chuckling like a potty mouthed 8 year old, then tell them you want **VERY** thin slices, not regular thickness.

- *MARINARA:* No, you don't have to use my marinara recipe. Use whatever you want, as long as it's 0 points. Mine is fast, quick and pretty danged good though, for only taking 10-12 minutes.

- *LOW POINT BREADING:* Reminder.... Rice Krispie brand rice cereal is NOT gluten free. If you have gluten allergies, make sure to find a legit, gluten free cereal. I use it instead of bread crumbs, because 1 cup of crushed rice creal is 3 points and results in a little over 1/2 cup of crumbs. Normal bread crumbs will only give you 1/4 cup of crumbs for 3 points.

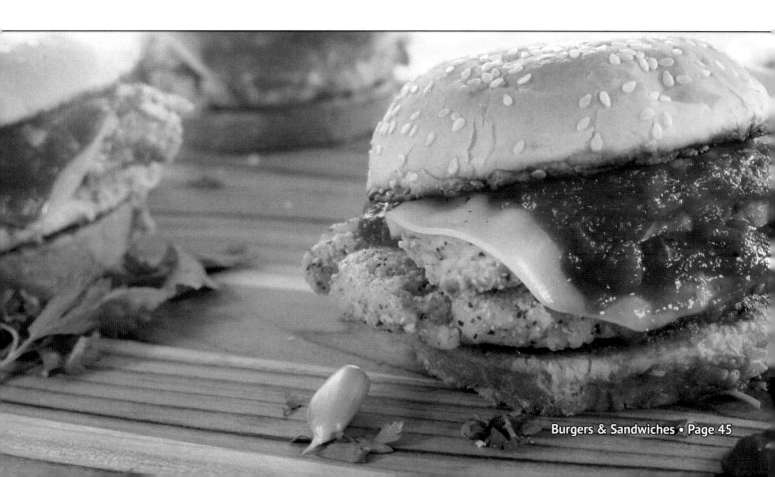

Chick-Fil-A copycat

This baby'll totally make you want to "Eat Mor Chikin".

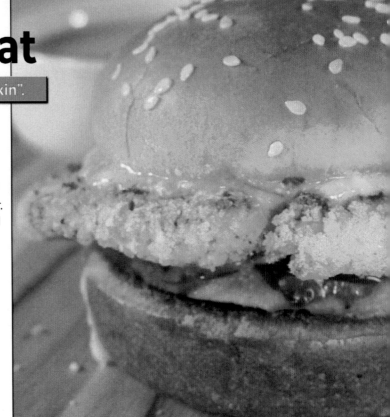

Full disclosure... the only reason that I made this sandwich was because I'm stuck home right now because of COVID. We're on lockdown and I'm rationing groceries. I realized that other than some jarred pickles, this sandwich uses NO produce. I just made a batch of my sauce for a video on Connect... It was one of those moments when the stars align and you end up with dinner.

A major reason that I'm happy to present this, my ww-erized version of their original sandwich, is because it will encourage people to try out my copycat sauce. A small "to go" packet of chick-fil-a sauce is 7 points. You can have an ENTIRE CUP of my low point version for half of that.

Servings Info.:
Yields: 4 sandwiches
Servings: 4
Serving Size: 1 sandwich

Points:	G	B	P
1 serving =	3	2	2
2 servings =	6	4	4
3 servings =	9	6	6
4 servings =	12	8	8

*(These listed points **DO NOT INCLUDE** the bun. Use whichever brand buns or bread you want, then add these points. These listed points are also for 5oz chicken breasts.)*

Ingredients:

Chicken: (see notes)
- 4 chicken breasts. If you're on the Green plan, only use chicken breasts that are 5oz or less, for 1 point each.

Chick-Fil-A copycat sauce:
- Prepare a batch of my "Chick Fil A" sauce, recipe on page 15.

Low Point Breading:
- 1 batch of my "Low Point Breading 2.0, from Cookbook 1, recipe on page 35, with the following changes:
    - If you are on the Green plan, use egg whites instead of whole eggs, to save points.
- Recipe can also be found/downloaded on my website, in the "Foundation Recipes" section.

Additional Ingredients:
- Dill pickle slices

Directions:

1. Prepare a batch of my low point breading 2.0, with the listed changes, if applicable. Set the dry ingredients in one shallow bowl and then beat the eggs (or egg whites) in another. Store the egg wash in the fridge, till ready.

2. Prepare the Chick-Fil-A sauce, set aside.

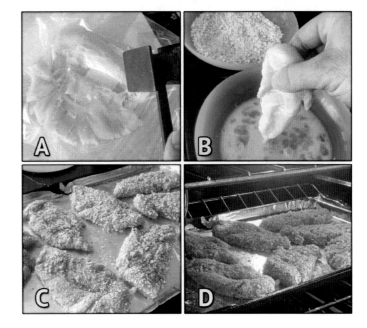

3. Preheat oven to 425 degrees. **(A)** Place chicken breasts in a gallon sized ziplock bag, then use a mallet or small pot to beat them silly. Flatten them down a little bit, for a more uniform thickness. **(B)** Dip each chicken breast into the egg wash, then into the crushed rice krispies breading mixture, lightly coating each side. **(C)** Place chicken on a foil lined pan, sprayed with cooking spray. Lightly spray the top of the chicken with cooking spray as well. **(D)** Bake the chicken for 12 minutes. Flip the chicken, then bake for another 8 minutes. Remove from oven and set aside.

4. While the chicken is in the oven, toast your hamburger buns or preferred bread.

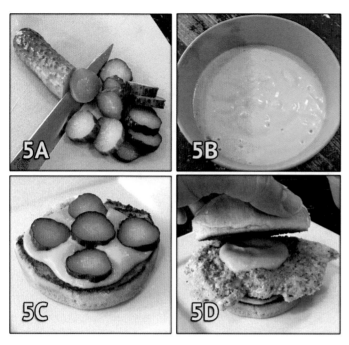

5. To assemble the sandwiches, first you must take your **(A)** dill pickle slices and **(B)** chick-fil-a sauce. **(C)** Smear a 1-1/2 Tbsp scoop of sauce onto the bottom bun, followed by some dill pickle slices. **(D)** Place one of the breaded chicken breasts on the pickles, followed by another dollop of sauce. Finally, top each sandwich with the toasted top bun. Done.

NOTES & SUGGESTIONS:

- **POINTS:** For folks on the Green plan, all proteins have points, therefore, I listed the use of 5oz chicken breasts. However, all of my Blue and Purple amigos can use any size chicken breasts they want. That's why the points go up 1 point on Green.
- **SAUCE:** The points for this recipe take into account that each sandwich gets 2 Tbsp of sauce on it. However, you can definitely use more sauce, if you'd like. Making a 1/2 batch of my copycat sauce only has a total of 3 points for an entire cup on Green and 2 total points for a cup on Blue. Just remember to halve all of the ingredients of the original recipe.
- **LOW POINT BREADING:** Reminder.... Rice Krispie brand rice cereal is NOT gluten free. If you have gluten allergies, make sure to find a legit, gluten free cereal. I use it instead of bread crumbs, because 1 cup of crushed rice cereal is 3 points and results in a little over 1/2 cup of crumbs. Normal bread crumbs will only give you 1/4 cup of crumbs for 3 points.
- **DRESS IT UP:** The original sandwich, available at all of their restaurants, is simply buttered buns with pickles and a breaded chicken breast. It's good, but plain-jane. Here, we're dressing it up with copycat chick-fil-a sauce, but you don't have to limit it to this. Feel free to add some lettuce, tomato, or a slice of low point cheese, such as Velveeta original, Borden's Fat Free cheddar slices, or Great Value cheese slices, all of which are 1 point for the first slice.

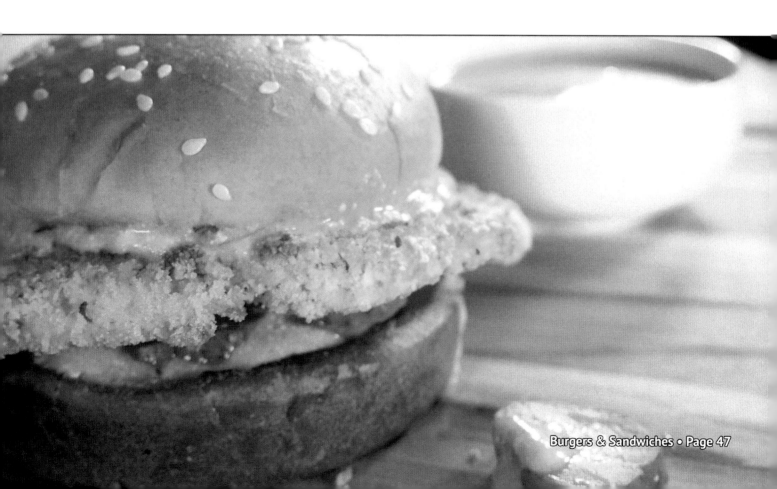

The Codfather

This simple sandwich'll make you an offer you can't refuse

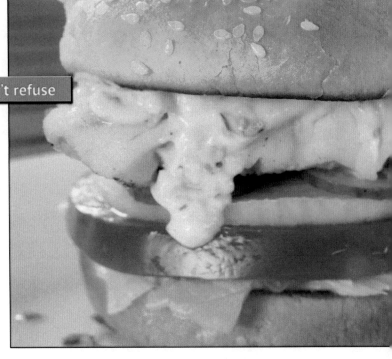

This is my nod to the kind of simple fish sandwich that you'd see on the menu at a mom 'n pop burger joint during Lent... or as I've dubbed it (Arnold Voice) ..."Da' Lentinator".

However, simple doesn't have to mean bland. So, this sandwich has a seared filet of cod, lightly seasoned and topped with a good sized dollop of my low point tartar sauce. Beneath it is a ton of fresh produce... thin sliced cucumbers, white onion, tomato, lettuce and another good dollop of tartar sauce. If you're looking for a quick and tasty sandwich, this will definitely hit the spot.

Servings Info.:
Yields: 4 sandwiches
Servings: 4
Serving Size: 1 sandwich

Points:

	G	B	P
1 serving =	2	0	0
2 servings =	4	1	1
3 servings =	6	1	1
4 servings =	7	2	2

(These listed points __DO NOT INCLUDE__ the bun. Use whichever brand buns or bread you want, then add these points. These listed points are also for 5oz of chicken.)

Ingredients:

Fish Filets: *(see notes)*
- 4 fresh, or previously frozen Cod filets. 4oz each**

Tartar Sauce:
- 1/2 batch of my low point Tartar sauce, recipe in Cookbook 2, on page 26.

Additional Ingredients:
- Fresh lettuce, any variety you prefer.
- 4 slices of tomato
- 4 thin slices of onion
- 16 thin slices of cucumber (4 per sandwich).

Directions:

1. Prepare a batch of my low point tartar sauce, set side.

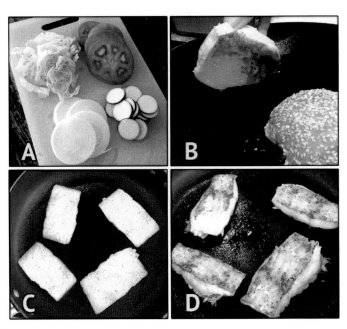

2. **(A)** Prep your veggies for a nice picture, then set aside. Pat cod filets dry with paper towels, then season with salt and pepper. Spray them with cooking spray and set aside. **(B)** Heat a large pan over medium heat for 1 minute, till hot. Place your buns (your **BURGER** buns!!) face down onto the pan till they are toasted. Set aside. **(C)** Spray the pan with cooking spray, then place the cod into the pan. Crank the heat up to medium-high and don't touch the fish. Cook for 3-4 minutes. **(D)** Spray the top of the fish with cooking spray, then use a spatula to get under the filets and flip them carefully. Cook for an additional 3-4 minutes. Remove from heat.

3. To assemble the sandwiches, **(A)** place a heaping Tablespoon of tartar sauce onto the bottom bun, **(B)** followed by some lettuce, a slice of tomato, then one of the onions slices. **(C)** Arrange 4 of the thin cucumber slices on top of the onion, followed by one of the cod filets and a good sized dollop of tartar sauce. **(D)** Finally, place the top bun on top of the sandwich. Done.

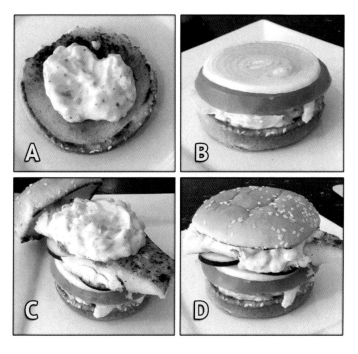

NOTES & SUGGESTIONS:

- *POINTS:* The listed points take into account the use of 1/4 cup of my low point tartar sauce, per sandwich. On blue & purple, 1/4 cup of my sauce is 0 points. On Green, it's 1 point per 1/4 cup serving. Other than the tartar sauce, this recipe has NO POINTS on blue & purple (of course, this doesn't count the buns.)
- *CHEESE:* Feel free to add cheese, if you want. I'm the Scrooge McDuck of smart points, so I didn't put any on my sandwiches.
- *TARTAR SAUCE:* Of course, you don't haaaaaave to use my low point tartar sauce recipe, but if you don't, remember to adjust your points accordingly.
- *CUCUMBERS:* Not everyone likes 'em, so they are optional. You could add some dill pickle slices for a nice tangy crunch.
- *FISH:* I realize that Cod is on the pricier side of white fish varieties. You can make this sandwich using ANY type of fish that you want. It'd be just as good with Tilapia, Salmon, Halibut, absolutely anything. You may need to adjust your cooking times, because some types of fish cook faster than others... and you don't want overcooked, dried out fish. Unless you're making fish jerky, but that's a different recipe.

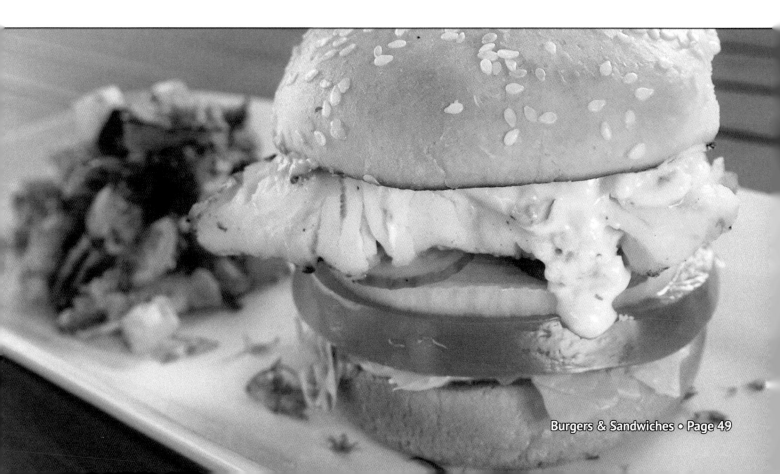

Crispy Fish Sandwich

My copycat WW-ified version of Wendy's Cod Sandwich

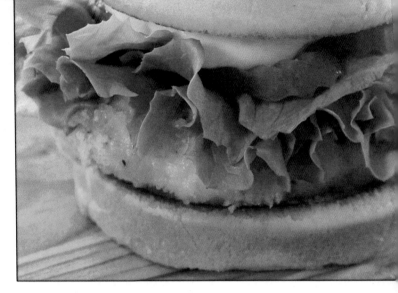

I... love... fish sandwiches. My absolute favorite fast food one has always been the Wendy's premium cod fish sandwich. It's simple, no frills and delicious. The actual version from the drive thru has 13 points and 21 grams of fat. Instead of a deep fried, processed fish filet, my recipe calls for breading and baking a cod filet with my low point breading recipe, then preparing a half batch of my low point tartar sauce, found in Cookbook 2. This recipe gives you all of the flavor and none of the guilt. Hey... not a bad tag line.

Servings Info.:	Points:	G	B	P
Yields: 4 sandwiches	1 serving =	3	1	1
Servings: 4	2 servings =	5	3	3
Serving Size: 1 sandwich	3 servings =	8	4	4
	4 servings =	10	5	5

(These listed points __DO NOT INCLUDE__ the bun. Use whichever brand buns or bread you want, then add these points. These listed points are also for 4-5oz cod filets.)

Ingredients:

Fish:
• 4 (4-5oz) cod filets, fresh or previously frozen.

Tartar Sauce:
• 1/2 batch of my low point tartar sauce. Recipe found in my Cookbook: Volume 2, on pg. 26.

Breading:
• 1 batch of my low point "breading 2.0", recipe in my Cookbook: Volume 1", on pg. 35, with the following changes:
   - Add 1/2 tsp old bay seasoning, if desired.
   - GREENIES!!! Use egg whites instead of whole eggs!

Additional Ingredients:
• Dill pickle slices, also called dill pickle "chips".
• Fresh green leaf lettuce

Directions:

1. Prepare a 1/2 batch of my tartar sauce recipe. Cover and set aside in the fridge.

2. Prepare a batch of my low point breading 2.0, with the listed changes. Set the dry ingredients in one shallow bowl and then beat the eggs (or 2 egg whites, if you're on the Green plan) in another bowl. Store the egg wash in the fridge, till ready to make the dish.

3. Preheat over to 425 degrees, line a pan with foil and spray with cooking spray. Set aside.

4. First things first... use paper towels to pat dry the cod filets. Seriously, sandwich each of the filets between paper towels and press. You want to get as much extra water out of them as possible. Soggy breading sucks.

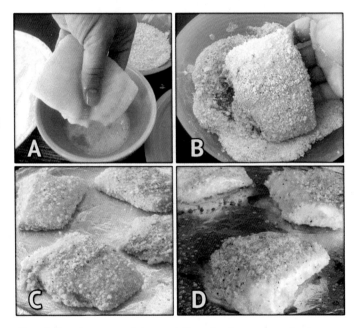

5. **(A)** Dredge one of the cod filets in the egg wash, then lift it out of the egg wash and wait a few seconds, so that some of the excess egg drips off. **(B)** Place the filet into the bowl with the crumbs, use your "dry" hand to coat both sides of the fish, then **(C)** place it on the foil lined pan. Repeat till all of the filets are breaded. Spray the tops of the breaded fish with cooking spray, then place in the preheated oven. **(D)** Bake at 425 degrees for 22 minutes. WHAT!?!?!? 22 minutes??? Hey, Karen... this is my recipe, just roll with it!

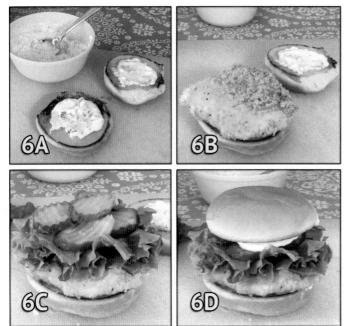

6A 6B 6C 6D

NOTES & SUGGESTIONS:

- *POINTS:* As noted, the listed points do not include buns. Also, for you folks on the Green plan, I used (4) 5 ounce cod filets. The listed points also take into account the breading, as well as the points from the tartar sauce, including the additional points that you Greenies get from the yogurt.
- *FISH:* Though I used Cod in my recipe, you can substitute it for any firm white fish that you'd like. I understand that cod's on the pricier side, in some areas.
- *Filet o' Fish?:* Remove the lettuce and pickles, then add 1 slice of low point American cheese on top of the filet, then BAM... low point copycat McDonald's fish filet sandwich, for just 1 additional point.
- *DRESSING:* Though my tartar sauce recipe is the bomb... I know that not everyone wants to make it (you savages!). Feel free to use any tartar sauce you want, or you can even use.... *gags*, ketchup. If you do use store bought tartar sauce or ketchup, remember to adjust your points. Also, please mail me back that friendship bracelet... because we're no longer BFF's.

6. To assemble the sandwiches, toast the buns, then **(A)** spread some of the tartar sauce onto each bun. I found that the sandwich tasted better when there was a bigger dollop on the top bun. **(B)** Place a baked cod filet onto the bottom bun, then **(C)** top the cod with some lettuce, followed by dill pickle slices. I used 5 dill pickle "chips" on my sandwich. **(D)** Finally, top the sandwich with the top bun. Done.

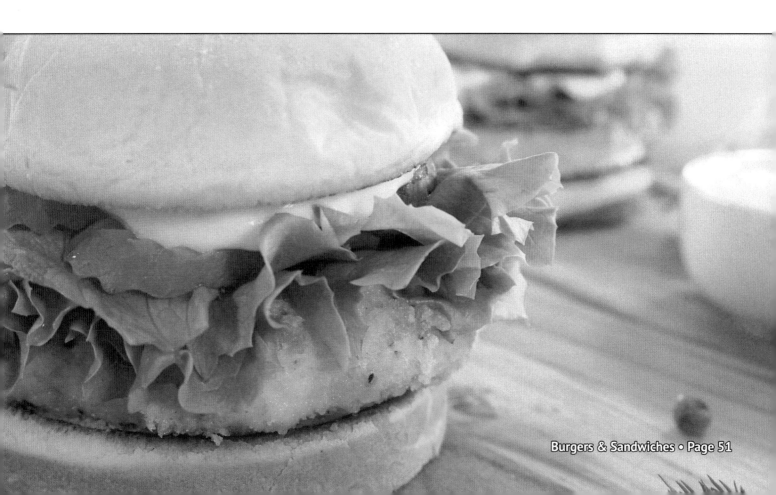

Enchilada Burger

Kind of like a "drowned" enchilada, but in burger form

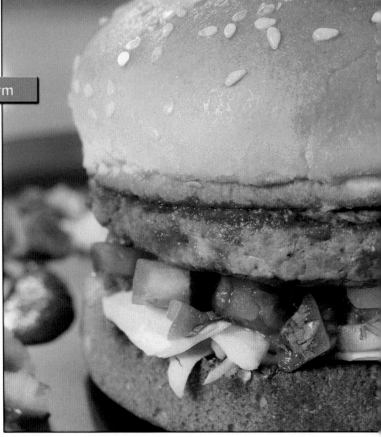

The thought for this burger came from one of those "what am I going to do with these leftovers?" days. I was trying to revise my old red enchilada sauce recipe, because I didn't realize that my original recipe, posted in Cookbook 1, was so hot that it'd burn paint off of a wall. Helpful Tip: When you buy CHEAP spices from the dollar store, like I do, the chili powder is a looooot more mild than regular brands like McCormick.

So, now that I suddenly had a leftover pot of newly made enchilada sauce in my fridge... and 2 kids that won't eat red enchiladas, I needed to figure out something to do with it. You're welcome... and sorry for melting your faces for a year and a half with my old ultra spicy red sauce recipe.

Servings Info.:

Yields: 4 burgers
Servings: 4
Serving Size: 1 burger

Points:

	G	B	P
1 serving =	1	0	0
2 servings =	2	0	0
3 servings =	3	0	0
4 servings =	4	0	0

*(These listed points **DO NOT INCLUDE** the bun. Use whichever brand buns or bread you want, then add these points. The listed points are for 2-3oz patties, for Greenies).*

Ingredients:

Burger Patties: *(see notes)*
- 1/2 batch mix of my "Savory" ground turkey, recipe in my "Cookbook: Volume 1", pg. 30.

Quick Enchilada Sauce: *(makes 3 cups, 0 points total)*
- 15oz tomato sauce
- 1-1/2 cups chicken broth
- 1-1/2 tsp garlic powder
- 1-1/2 tsp onion powder
- 1-1/2 tsp cumin
- 1 to 2 tsp chili powder (to taste, some brands are spicier).
- 1/4 tsp salt

Pico De Gallo:
- 1 cup diced tomato (1 large tomato)
- 3/4 cup diced onion
- 1 Tbsp chopped/diced, canned green chiles. (I used mild, I'm a wimp)**
- 1/2 cup finely chopped fresh cilantro
- 2 Tbsp lime juice
- 1/4 to 1/2 tsp salt, to taste

Additional Ingredients:
- Shredded cabbage
- 2-1/2 Tbsp plain fat free Greek yogurt, mixed with 1 Tbsp water, and 1 tsp lemon juice. Set aside (makes a sour cream-ish sauce).
- Additional fresh cilantro

Directions:

1. Combine all of the Enchilada sauce ingredients in a small pot. Bring to a boil over medium heat, reduce heat, then simmer for 5 minutes. Turn off heat, set aside.

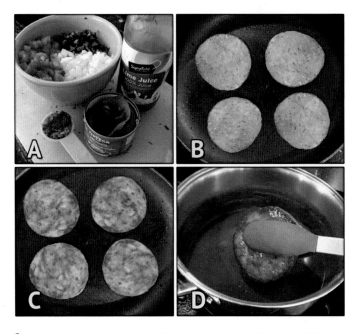

2. **(A)** Mix the ingredients for the pico de gallo, set aside. **(B)** After the "savory" ground turkey rests for 20 minutes, wet your hands and form the meat into 4 patties. Preheat a pan on medium heat for 1 minute, spray with cooking spray, then cook patties for 2 minutes. **(C)** Flip the patties and cook for an additional 2 minutes. **(D)** Place the burger patties into the pot of warm/hot enchilada sauce.

3. When all the burgers are in the sauce, toast your hamburger buns or preferred bread.

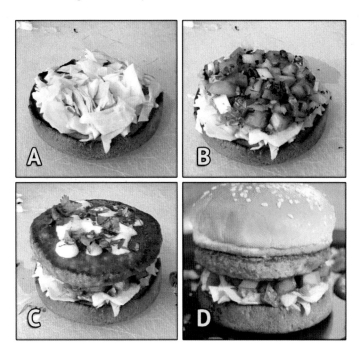

4. To assemble the burger, **(A)** place a mound of shredded cabbage onto the bottom bun, **(B)** followed by a 1/4 cup scoop of the pico de gallo. **(C)** Carefully use some kitchen tongs to take one burger patty out of the enchilada sauce and set it onto the pico de gallo. Drizzle the patty with a bit of the thinned Greek yogurt, a little more enchilada sauce, and a sprinkle of fresh chopped cilantro. **(D)** Finally, top each sandwich with the toasted top bun. Done.

NOTES & SUGGESTIONS:

- *ENCHILADA SAUCE:* Here's a cool thing... You don't have to make mine. I encourage it, but you don't have too. If you use regular canned, low fat red enchilada sauce, yes it's high in points, but that's for a good sized serving of sauce. When you dunk the patties in the sauce, you're only really coating them in maybe 1 to 1-1/2 Tbsp of sauce. So, depending on the brand you buy and the amount you use, the canned sauce maaaay also be 0 points per burger. Scan the cans and do the math, but... making mine eliminates the hassle.
- *PICO DE GALLO:* I am a spicy food sissy. Seriously, I think the mild sauce at Taco Bell has kick, which is why I used canned, mild green chiles, instead of the traditional jalapeño peppers. If you'd like to use jalapeños, feel free. I'll be over here chugging a gallon of milk. Also, to save time, you can purchase ready made pico de gallo at your grocery store. It can usually be found in the produce department.
- *CHEESE:* Though enchiladas normally have cheese, ok... ALWAYS have cheese... I didn't add any to these burgers. It's a known fact that I'm the Scrooge McDuck of points. If you'd like to add some cheese, feel free, but adjust your points.
- *POINTS:* Even though the "filling" for these burgers is 0 points per serving, on Blue & Purple... for the love of God, use that coconut on your neck. 0 points doesn't mean 0 calories. The only points for your burgers are going to be for your buns. That does NOT mean that you should gorge and eat 4 burgers. When you prepare and eat an ultra low point meal, you MUST be even more responsible and mindful of how much food you eat, even more than your amgios eating high point foods and trying to eat enough to get blue dots. Eat 1 burger and be content. Don't eat 3 or 4 low point burgers simply because you have points, that defeats the purpose of cooking like this.

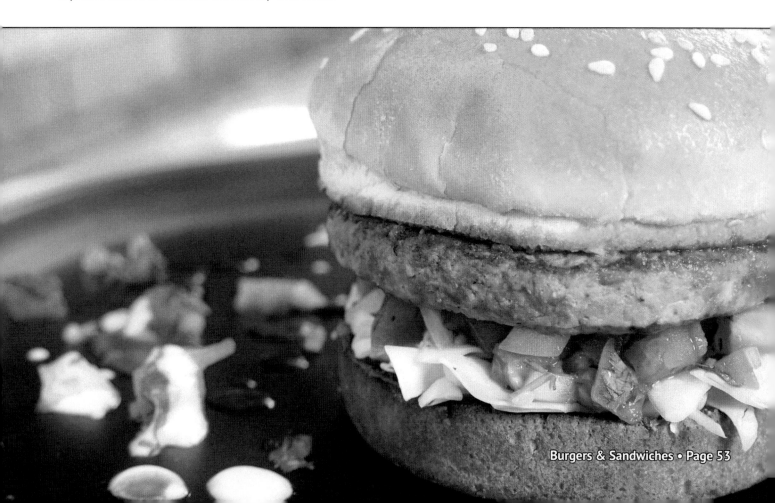

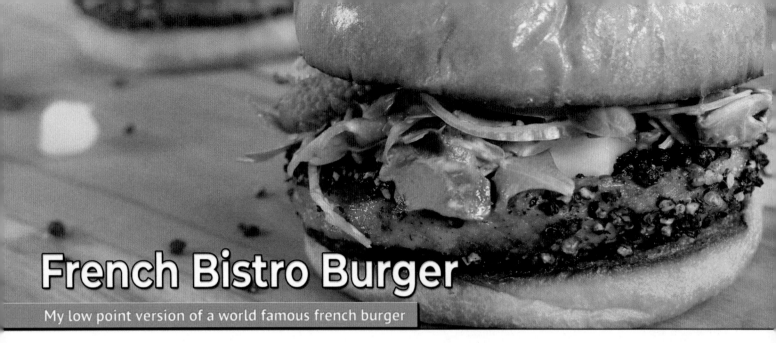

French Bistro Burger

My low point version of a world famous french burger

When I was trying to find inspiration pictures for a suuuuper fancy & swanky burger, I stumbled upon multiple articles, that ALL referenced a cheeseburger from a French restaurant in Manhattan. Multiple world acclaimed publications have all dubbed it "the greatest cheeseburger in America". The original version is a high end burger full of French attitude. It has a beef brisket patty, crusted in black pepper, with a thick slab of French triple cream cheese, dressed arugula, french mini pickles, and thin sliced red onion. It's then served with a pan sauce made with cognac and heavy cream. THIS is my lighter version.

Ingredients:

"Au Poivre" Burger Patties
- 1 lb batch of my "savory" ground turkey. Recipe in my "Cookbook: Volume 1" on page 30.
- Coarse ground black pepper (as much as you want)

Dijon Vinaigrette:
- 2-1/2 Tbsp plain fat free Greek yogurt
- 1 Tbsp dijon mustard
- 1 tsp olive oil
- 2 tsp white wine vinegar

Au Poivre Pan Sauce:
- 1 Tbsp water
- 3 Tbsp Brandy (see notes)**
- 1-1/2 tsp cornstarch
- 1/2 cup plain unsweetened almond milk
- salt and pepper to taste

Additional Toppings:
- 6 pieces mini Babybel Light cheese (see notes)**
- 5 oz baby arugula
- THIIIIIIIN sliced red onion
- Cornichons, also known as Gherkins. They're jarred and located by the pickles and olives at the grocery store. They're lil pickles.

Directions:

1. Prepare the batch of "savory" meat, cover, set aside.

2. Remove the red wax covers from the Babybel cheese, **(A)** then put them in a microwave safe bowl. **(B)** heat for 20 seconds at a time, till melted together. Set aside.

Servings Info.:	Points:	G	B	P
Yields: 4 burgers	1 serving =	5	3	3
Servings: 4	2 servings =	10	6	6
Serving Size: 1 burger	3 servings =	15	9	9
	4 servings =	20	12	12

(These listed points DO NOT INCLUDE the bun. Use whichever brand buns or bread you want, then add these points. This is what's between the buns)

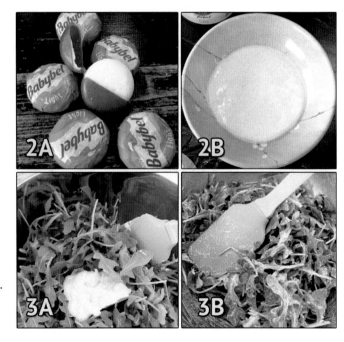

3. Now, let's dress the arugula! Mix together the Greek yogurt, dijon, olive oil and vinegar until smooth. **(A)** Add the arugula and dressing into a mixing bowl, **(B)** then toss to combine. Set aside.

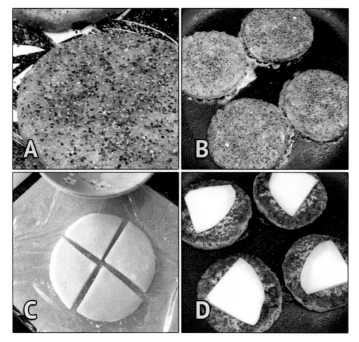

- *PATTIES:* Though my fancy pictures use large cracked black peppercorns... I do noooooot recommend it. The burgers are ridiculously spicy like that. I had to remake them with smaller sized cracked pepper. Use a pepper mill, or buy a small, inexpensive container of coarse ground black pepper from the store. Use as much as you want.
    * Cook the patties with cooking spray. I also used 1 tsp of I Can't Believe It's Not Butter Light, because it's 0 points. I used 99% fat free ground turkey, so it cooks very fast, hence the 2 minutes per side.
- *VINAIGRETTE:* If you're allergic to Dairy, you can use silken tofu in place of the Greek. Also, I only used 2-1/2 Tbsp of Greek yogurt so that it would stay 0 points for Greenies. Also, if you don't have white wine vinegar, distilled white vinegar will work too, it just won't sound as fancy.
- *PAN SAUCE:* Same thing. If you're allergic to nuts, honestly.. you don't need to ask what to use. Use whatever you want, just adjust your points accordingly.
- *BRANDY:* The traditional recipe uses expensive cognac. I decided to use brandy, because you can get a small 100ml bottle, for $2.50, from pretty much any small liquor store. Don't want to use alcohol? Use some beef broth instead. It won't be the same, but it'll have a rich, peppery, beefy gravy in its place. That'll still taste pretty good.
- *CHEESE:* I used mini Babybel Light cheese, because most everyone can get it at most major grocery stores. The 6 pieces have 8 points. A good substitution would be 3oz of goat cheese, same points. Or, use 8 points of any cheese.

4. **(A)** Form the raw meat into 4 patties, liberally coat both sides of the patties with a good amount of cracked pepper. **(B)** Heat a pan for a minute over medium heat, then add the patties. Cook for 2 minutes. **(C)** During that 2 minutes, take the cheese out of the bowl and slice into 4 pieces. **(D)** Flip the burgers and place a cheese quarter on each patty. Pour 2-3 Tbsp of water into the pan, cover with a lid and cook for 2 more minutes. Remove the patties, turn off the flame.

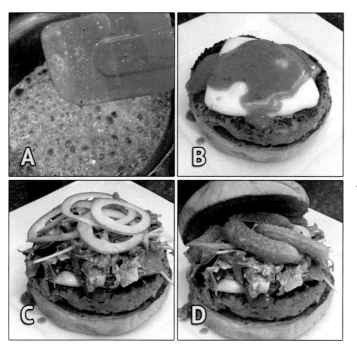

5. To make the pan sauce, **(A)** Mix the pan sauce ingredients in a cup, till smooth, then pour into the hot pan. Turn the flame back on to high and bring to a simmer. Stir for 1-2 minutes, till starting to thicken. Pour into a cup and set aside. **(B)** Toast your burger buns, then place your patty onto the bottom bun and scoop a good spoonfull of hot sauce onto the cheese. **(C)** Place a mound of the arugula onto the burger, followed by a few of the thin sliced red onions. **(D)** Lastly, slice a few of the thin pickles in half, lengthwise, then place them on top. Done.

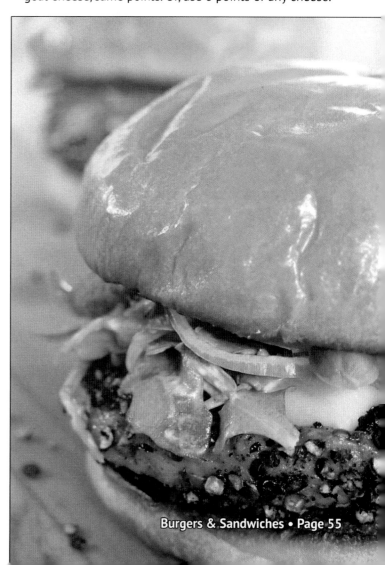

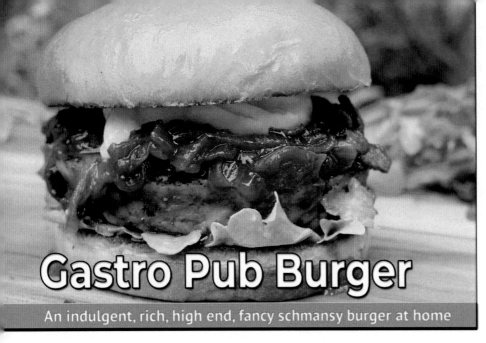

Gastro Pub Burger

An indulgent, rich, high end, fancy schmansy burger at home

A Gastro Pub is just a fancy name for a bar/cafe that serves small portions of high priced, snooty sounding food. Why pay the cost of a house payment for one of their fancy burgers, when you can make one at home? This baby has a 1/4lb 'savory' turkey patty with a slice of smoked gouda... smoky bacon jam, dressed arugala and a poached egg on top for a luxuriously runny yolk.

All of the flavors are awesome. When combined, you get the thick, meaty patty with the smoky gouda cheese. The sweet, tangy, smoky onion and bacon reduction, the poached egg that oozes rich, creamy and fatty yolk onto the burger... and all that richness gets balanced by the citrusy lemon dressing and peppery arugala.

Servings Info.:
Yields: 4 burgers
Servings: 4
Serving Size: 1 burger

Points:

	G	B	P
1 serving =	6	2	2
2 servings =	13	5	5
3 servings =	19	7	7
4 servings =	25	9	9

(Greenies have a TON more points, because of the 1lb of turkey and 4 whole eggs.)

Ingredients:

Burger Patties:
• 1 lb batch of my "Savory" ground turkey mix, formed into (4) 1/4 pound patties. Recipe in my "Cookbook: Volume 1", on pg. 30.

Lemon Dijon Dressing:
• 2 Tbsp fat free plain Greek yogurt
• 1 Tbsp lemon juice
• 1 Tbsp dijon mustard
• 1/4 tsp olive oil
• 1/8 tsp each, salt and pepper
• 1/4 tsp 0 point sweetener o' choice

Smoky Red Onion & Bacon Jam:
• 4 points worth of turkey bacon (see notes)
• 2 large red onions, halved and sliced thin.
• 1-1/2 cups beef broth (scan to ensure it's 0 points)
• 2 Tbsp apple cider vinegar
• 1/4 tsp salt
• 1/4 tsp black pepper
• 1 tsp 0 point brown sugar substitute, OR 1 tsp regular sweetener plus 1/4 tsp molasses.
• 1/2 tsp smoked paprika
• 1/2 tsp unsweetened cocoa powder
• 2 tsp balsamic vinegar
• 1-2 Tbsp sugar free syrup (pancake syrup). Scan the brands, some give you 1 Tbsp for 0 points, some allow 2 Tbsp.

Additional Ingredients:
• 4 slices smoked gouda, thin sliced (see notes).
• Fresh arugula
• 4 large eggs

Directions:

1. Prepare the meat mixture and patties, set aside.

2. Mix the Dressing ingredients together till smooth, toss with the arugala, cover and set aside.

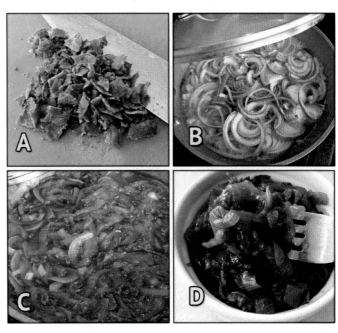

3. **(A)** Cook all of the bacon in a large pan, with cooking spray, till crisp. Remove from pan and chop into small pieces. Set aside. **(B)** To the same pan, add the sliced red onions, 3/4 cup beef broth, apple cider vinegar, salt, pepper and brown sugar substitute or sweetener and molasses. Bring to a simmer, cover and cook for 15 minutes. **(C)** After 15 minutes, add the remaining 3/4 cup beef broth, smoked paprika, cocoa powder, balsamic vinegar and syrup. Cover and simmer on medium-low for another 15-20 minutes, till **(D)** it resembles a thick jam. Add more salt and pepper, if desired.

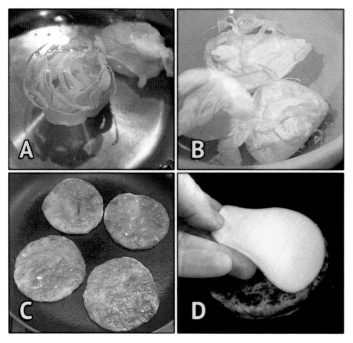

4. **(A)** While the jam is cooking, bring a medium pot of water to a low boil, just to where it's starting to bubble. Add a little bit of vinegar into the water, then stir to create a whirlpool effect. Gently place the raw eggs into the water, it doesn't matter if the egg whites "feather out", we won't be using those anyways. Let the eggs cook in the low boiling water for 3 minutes. **(B)** Remove the eggs with a slotted spoon, and place in a bowl of cool water. Set aside. **(C)** Preheat a large pan for 1 minute over medium heat, then cook burger patties for 2 minutes and flip. **(D)** Place a slice of gouda on each patty, cook 2 more minutes. Done.

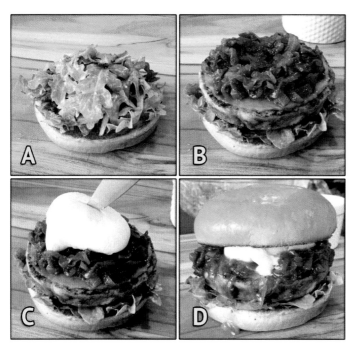

5. **(A)** Toast your sandwich buns o' choice, then place a mound of dressed arugala onto the bottom bun. **(B)** Set a burger patty on top of the arugala, followed by a 1/4 cup scoop of the red onion bacon jam. **(C)** Make a small crater in the center of the onion jam and place a poached egg on top. Make a small slit in the egg. **(D)** Place the top bun over the egg, gently push down to squeeze out some yolk. Done.

NOTES & SUGGESTIONS:

- ***BACON JAM:*** This one is a bit tricky. Use WHATEVER type of bacon you want, but use no more than 4 points worth. Depending on your brand, you may get more than others. Oscar Mayer turkey bacon is 5 points for 4 slices, where Trader joes uncured turkey bacon lets you have 4 slices for 1 point. Use as much as you can, of whatever brand or type you want, but don't go over 4 points.
  - * ***Sweeteners:*** As stated, you can use either regular sweetener with 1/4 tsp molasses added to it, or use 0 point brown sugar substitute... your choice. Heck, if you want, use regular brown sugar and regular maple syrup... but adjust your points.
- ***THIN SLICED SMOKED GOUDA???:*** To get thin sliced smoked gouda, you'll need to go to your grocery store's deli department. Ask them to slice you some smoked gouda, AS THIN AS THEY CAN MAKE IT. When they sliced it for me, I took it home, weighed the slices, and they were each around 10 grams in weight, making the first slice 1 point, the 2nd slice 3 points, the 3rd slice 4 points and the 4th slice 6 points. The deli-guy informed me that the setting he used, was pretty much the universal "thinnest" setting they can slice cheese at with most grocery store deli cutters.
- ***POACHED EGGS:*** Want to eliminate the hassle of poaching the eggs? No problem. Fry your eggs instead, just make sure to keep the egg yolks runny. It's a lot less work if you choose to fry the eggs... but it's not as food-snooty.
- ***PATTY POINTS:*** You can lower the burgers 1 point, on the Green plan, by making thinner 2oz patties.

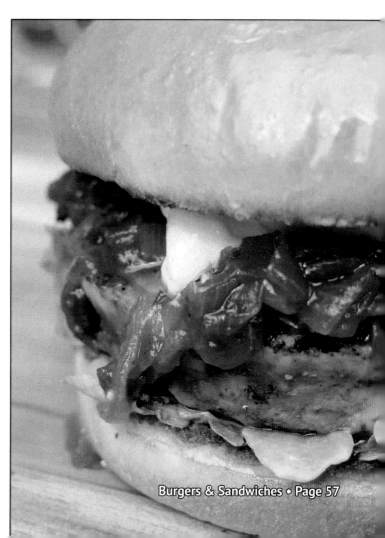

Green Chile Chorizo

My take on a delicious, New Mexico classic

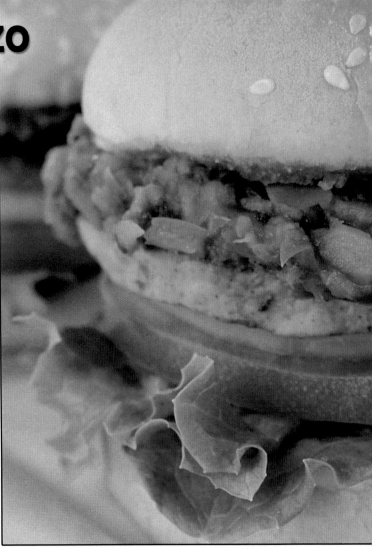

Let's start off by addressing the elephant in the room, this is NOT 100% authentic. You southwest folks need to come to terms with the fact that not everyone can get "Hatch" chiles. This recipe is prepared in the same way as a normal Hatch chile recipe, but using whatever peppers you have available. In my case, I used Anaheim peppers, which are the same as Ortega peppers. You can also use Poblanos. Anaheim and Poblanos are NOT very spicy, they are maybe 2/10 on the spicy scale. They have a delicious subtle smoky flavor that is enhanced by charring them in the oven. Spice it up with the addition of a Jalapeno or hot sauce.

Servings Info.:
Yields: 4 burgers
Servings: 4
Serving Size: 1 burger

Points:

	G	B	P
1 serving =	1	0	0
2 servings =	2	0	0
3 servings =	3	0	0
4 servings =	4	0	0

(These listed points DO NOT INCLUDE the bun. Use whichever brand buns or bread you want, then add these points. This is what's between the buns)

Ingredients:

Ground Turkey Chorizo Patties
- 1/2 batch of my ground turkey "Chorizo", recipe in my "Cookbook: Volume 1" on page 27. (Halve the recipe).
- Mix 1 Tablespoon of fat free plain greek yogurt into the raw meat mixture, for added moisture.
- Reduce the chili powder to 2 teaspoons, instead of 3.

Green Chile Spread:
- 5 good sized Anaheim Chiles. *(see notes**)*
- 1 small red onion, sliced
- 2 medium cloves garlic

Additional Toppings:
- Onion, thin sliced
- Tomato slices
- Lettuce, any preferred variety.

Spread:
- 3 Tbsp fat free plain Greek yogurt
- 1/4 tsp each chipotle chili powder and cumin
- Hot sauce to taste

Directions:

1. First things first, the meat. Mix up a 1/2 batch of my ground turkey chorizo, then cover it with plastic wrap and let it sit for 20 minutes. Once it's rested, move it to a cutting board and form into a ball. If the meat is a little tacky, lightly spray it with cooking spray to make it easier to manage.

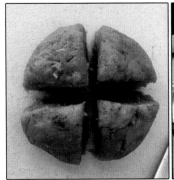 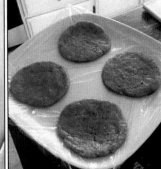

2. Slice the meat into 4 equal sections., then form each of the sections into patties. Set aside to allow the flavors to continue melding, as you prepare the rest of the ingredients.

3. Preheat oven to 450 degrees. Line a baking pan with foil paper and spray with cooking spray. Place the garlic cloves into a small pouch of foil, then spray the garlic with cooking spray and close the pouch. Place the sliced onions next to the pouch.

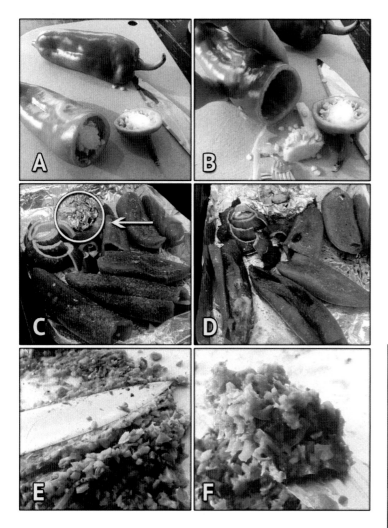

- For the peppers.. USE WHATEVER PEPPERS YOU WANT! If you have access to Hatch chiles, use those. If you want a milder chile, use Anahiem or poblanos. Want a little extra kick? Add a Jalapeño. Also, you don't HAVE to remove the seeds and membrane, like I did in steps 4A and 4B. Leaving them in will make your mixture spicier.
- Feel free to add a slice of cheese, I forgot to put it on. 🍺
- Reminder, the points listed do NOT take into account a bun. This way, you can use whatever buns or bread you want, then just add these points to it.
- I roasted my chiles in the oven, rather than charring them on a grill, because a lot of people don't have a gas grill, or they don't want to stink up their house by charring peppers directly on their gas stovetop. If you want to use either of those 2 methods, have at it. I have to make my recipes as accessible to people as possible.
- You can use larger 1/4 pound patties, but adjust points if if you're on the green plan.

4. Ok, you traditionalists... get over it, this is how I do it.
   (A) Slice the top ends off of the peppers, to expose the seeds and membranes, that's where all of the heat is. **(B)** I have nooo heat tolerance, so I removed most of the seeds and membranes. **(C)** Place the peppers onto the foil lined pan, along with the onions and foil pouch with the garlic in it (circled). **(D)** Roast at 450 for 20 minutes, then remove from the oven. *(optional) You can peel the skin from the peppers if you want, but I didn't... I'm lazy and hungry.*
   (E) Use a knife to finely chop all of the onions, chiles and garlic. Occasionally press down on them with your knife blade, to smash the peppers and make a nice "mash".
   (F) Season with a little salt and pepper or cumin, to taste.

5. For the spread, mix the Greek yogurt, chipotle chili powder, cumin and hot sauce (to taste), till well combined. Set aside.

6. To assemble the burgers, first... toast your buns, then smear with a little bit of the Greek yogurt/hot sauce spread. Second, place some of the lettuce onto the bottom bun, then a slice of tomato, followed by a thin sliced of onion. Place a chorizo patty on top of the onion, then dollop a nice scoop of the green chili mixture onto the patty. Finally, cover with the top bun and enjoy.

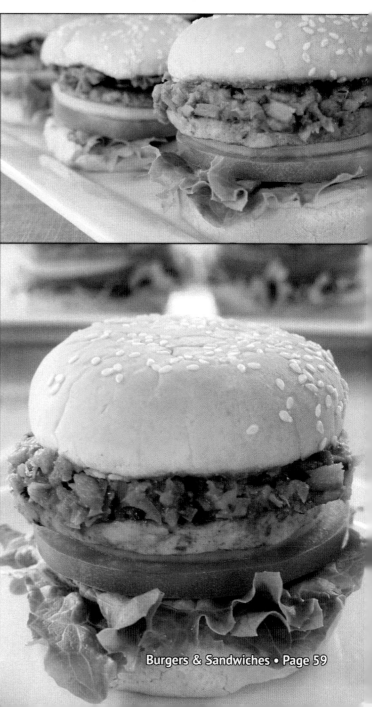

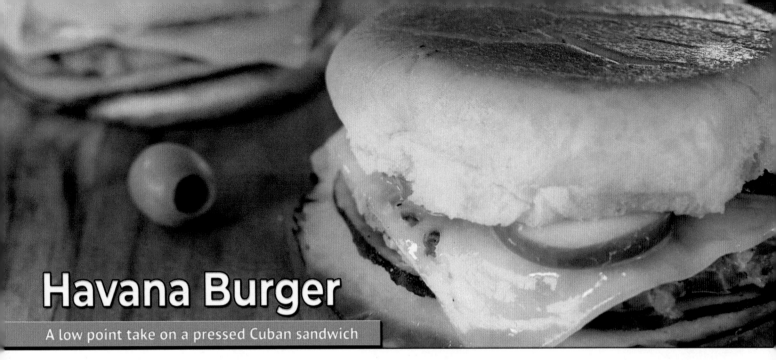

Havana Burger

A low point take on a pressed Cuban sandwich

A Cuban sandwich is traditionally a ham, pork & swiss cheese sandwich, with a mustard/mayo spread and pickles, that's toasted and pressed like a panini. I was looking up famous sandwiches, online, to try and make a burger versions of. When a Cuban sandwich popped up, I thought it'd be awesome to make a ww-ified burger version! What REALLY makes this baby pop is toasting/pressing the finished hamburger in the same fashion as a panini, to give a super crunchy bread crust. This is a great low point stand in for the original, but in burger form.

Ingredients:

Cuban Picadillo Burger Patties
- 1/2 batch of my ground turkey "Picadillo", recipe in my "Cookbook: Volume 1" on page 28. (Halve the recipe).
- Remove the raisins from the meat seasoning recipe.

Roasted Garlic Mustard Spread:
- 4 medium garlic cloves, still in skin.
- 6 Tbsp plain fat free Greek yogurt
- 2 Tbsp yellow mustard (like French's hot dog mustard)
- 2 tsp water
- pinch of salt and pepper

Additional Toppings:
- Dill pickle slices, as many as you want, the more the merrier.
- 4 slices light swiss cheese (see note)***
- 5 oz uncured, deli sliced ham (you want a brand that will give you 12 slices for 2 points).

Directions:

1. Prepare the 1/2 batch of meat, cover and set aside.

2. Now, let's roast some garlic, so that we can make the spread! Preheat your oven to 375 degrees. Slice the ends off of one side, from 4 cloves of garlic. Place the garlic into a small tin foil pouch, then coat with 0 point cooking spray. Close the pouch and cook at 375 degrees for 45 minutes. Let the garlic cool for 5 minutes. Squeeze the "back side" of the garlic, to remove the soft, roasted garlic.

Servings Info.:
Yields: 4 burgers
Servings: 4
Serving Size: 1 burger

Points:

	G	B	P
1 serving =	3	2	2
2 servings =	7	4	4
3 servings =	10	6	6
4 servings =	13	8	8

(These listed points DO NOT INCLUDE the bun. Use whichever brand buns or bread you want, then add these points. This is what's between the buns)

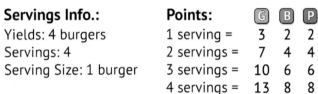

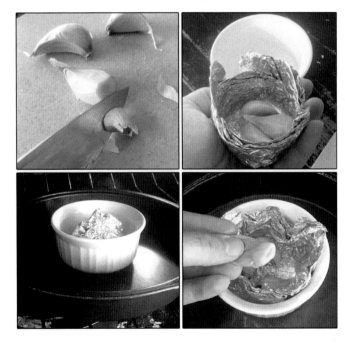

3. Place the Greek yogurt, yellow mustard and water into a bowl, stir to combine. Mash the garlic and mince with a knife, then mash again. Stir the mashed garlic into the yogurt/mustard. Season with a pinch of salt and pepper, cover and set aside.

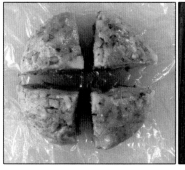 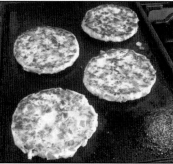

4. The meat will be a little tacky, hit it with cooking spray to take care of that. Section the meat into 4 sections, then form into patties and cook till browned on both sides.

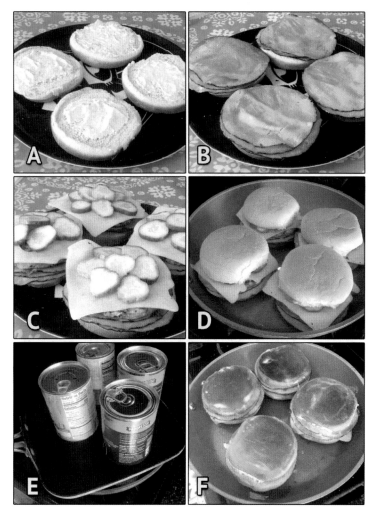

5. Now... let's assemble some Burger/Panini hybrids!!! First, start heating up a large pan over medium heat. **(A)** Spread 1 Tbsp of the garlic/mustard spread onto the bottom bun, **(B)** followed by 3 slices of ham. **(C)** Place a cooked turkey patty on top of the ham, followed by a slice of the cheese, then a good amount of pickle slices. Put another 1 Tbsp of spread on the top bun... then let's make some panini burgers. **(D)** Spray cooking spray into your hot pan, then transfer all of the burgers into it. **(E)** Place a large pan or or other metal surface on top of all of the burgers, then place cans or additional pots on top, to compress the burgers, just like you would to make a panini. **(F)** After 60 seconds, spray the top of the burgers with cooking spray, then carefully flip them and toast again. Enjoy.

NOTES & SUGGESTIONS:

- CHEESE: The listed points are dependent upon using 1 point per slice, reduced fat swiss cheese. If you can't find that, go to the deli counter at your grocery store and have them slice you some swiss cheese slices, VERY thin. Make sure to stress that you want them THIN, or they won't do it. If you have to use regular swiss slices, the burgers will go up 1 additional point each, which is still pretty dang low in points.
- You can eliminate steps D, E & F, by using a panini press or George Foreman grill to press/toast the burgers.
- Try to use thin sliced uncured ham, it's lowest in calories and points, typically. Weigh the ham when you get it home. You're aiming for 2 points for 5oz, which should give you 12 slices.
- Use whatever type of bun you want, but adjust your points accordingly.
- I'd recommend patting the vinegar off of the pickles.

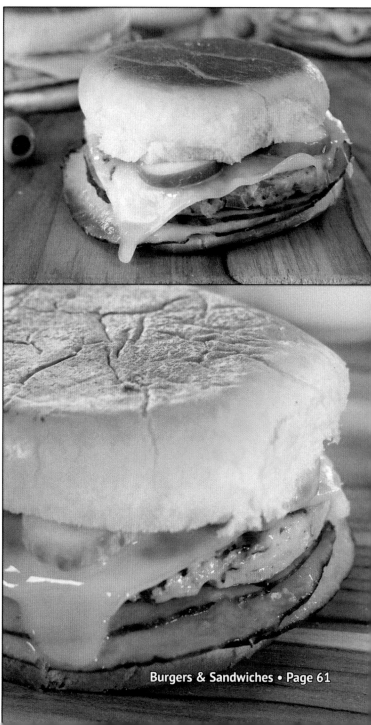

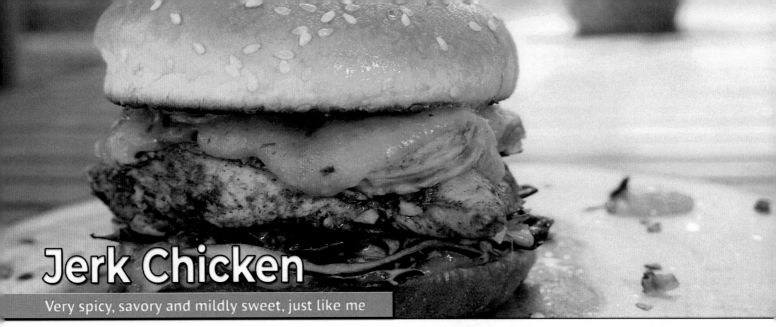

Jerk Chicken

Very spicy, savory and mildly sweet, just like me

No, I'm not insulting chickens. "Jerk" is an actual seasoning blend from the Caribbean, famously used in "Jerk Chicken". For this recipe, I wanted to try and use my ground meat "Jerk" seasoning recipe, as a marinade, rather than mixing it into ground meat. It makes for an insanely spicy, yet savory chicken breast. Traditional recipes are made with scotch bonnet peppers, but not everyone has access to those, so I'm using habaneros.

Servings Info.:
Yields: 4 sandwiches
Servings: 4
Serving Size: 1 sandwich

Points:

	G	B	P
1 serving =	1	0	0
2 servings =	2	0	0
3 servings =	3	0	0
4 servings =	4	0	0

(These listed points DO NOT INCLUDE the bun. Use whichever brand buns or bread you want, then add these points. These also account for using a 1 point, 2oz chicken breast for Greenies. If you want a larger chicken breast, adjust your points, if you're on the Green plan.)

Ingredients:

Jerk Seasoned Chicken Breasts
- 4 boneless, skinless chicken breasts. Greenies, keep them to no more than 1 point per piece, by weight.
- 1 batch of my "Jerk Seasoning" mix, recipe in my "Cookbook: Volume 1", on page 29. Make the following changes.
    - Use 2 medium cloves garlic, minced
    - Leave out the baking soda.
    - Leave out the chicken flavored bouillon.

Mango Chili Sauce - *(makes 1-1/4 cup, (5) 1/4 cup servings, 0 point)*
- 1 good sized ripe mango. Skinned, core removed, pureed. You should end up with around 1-1/4 cup pureed mango.
- 1 Tbsp asian garlic chili sauce, such as Huy Fung brand.
- 1 tsp 0 point sweetener o' choice.

Simple Slaw Dressing:
- 2-1/2 Tbsp fat free plain Greek yogurt
- 2 Tbsp apple cider vinegar
- 1/4 tsp salt
- 1/4 tsp black pepper
- 1 tsp 0 point sweetener o' choice.
- 1 tsp light mayonnaise

Additional Ingredients:
- 2 unripe bananas, sliced into 20 thick slices, around 1/2" thick. (not kidding, you want bananas that are somewhat green).
- 1/2 head red cabbage. Remove the core, then slice the head in half. Pretend you're a guillotine and it's the French revolution.

Directions:

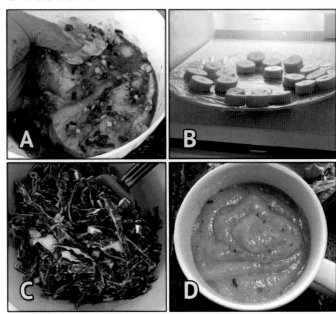

1. **(A)** Mix all of the marinade ingredients together. Coat the chicken breasts, cover, store for at LEAST one hour. **(B)** Cover a plate with plastic wrap, place banana slices on the plate, store in the freezer for later. **(C)** Mix all of the "simple slaw dressing" ingredients, till well mixed. Slice the cabbage and green onion, then mix with the dressing. Cover and set aside in the fridge. **(D)** Mix all of the ingredients together for the mango chili sauce. If you'd like your puree a little thinner, add some water. Set aside while the chicken marinates. The longer it marinates, the better.

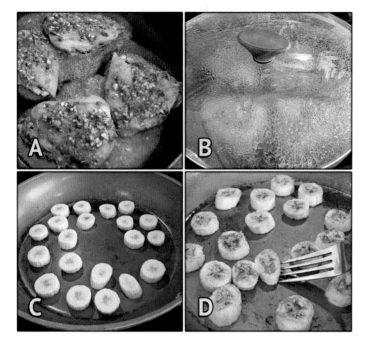

- **CHILI PEPPERS:** As stated before, traditional Jerk chicken marinade recipes, call for using Scotch Bonnet peppers. Not every store carries them, so I chose to use habanero peppers in my recipe. If you are able to get Scotch Bonnets... by all means, have at it. Remember, use gloves when handling the peppers.

- **MANGO CHILI SAUCE:** If you don't like Mango, feel free to customize the sauce by swapping it out for ANY fruit that you would like, such as pureed pineapple or peach. Also, pureed fruit gets points if you drink it, not if you use it as part of a dish that you'll be eating.

- **SLAW:** This is a very, very, very simple dressing. If you'd like to jazz it up a little bit, toast 1 tsp of sesame seeds in a hot pan for 2-3 minutes, or till lightly browned. 1tsp of sesame seeds is 1 point... but 1 tsp of TOASTED sesame seeds is 0 points in the WW database.

- **FROZEN BANANAS?:** Unless you freeze them first, they will turn to goop when you quick-sear them. If you are on the Purple plan, Plaintains are 0 points, use those instead. You don't need to freeze plaintains. On Green & Blue, if you use plaintains, it'll add 3 points per burger.

2. After your chicken has marinated for at least an hour, heat a large pan over medium-high heat for 1 minute. **(A)** Spray the pan with cooking spray and place the chicken and marinade into the pan. Cook for 2 minutes, then flip. **(B)** Cover the pan, reduce heat to medium-low, cook for 20 mins. Turn off heat, keep pan covered for 10 more minutes. **(C)** Heat a large pan over medium heat for 1 minute. Remove frozen banana slices from freezer. Spray with cooking spray, sear for 1 minute. **(D)** Spray the bananas with cooking spray again, then flip and sear for 1 more minute. Done.

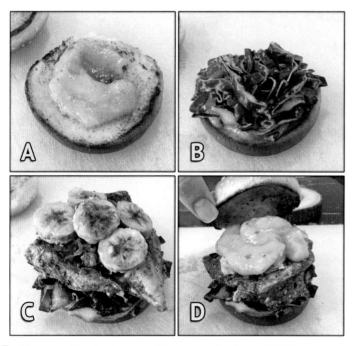

3. To assemble the burgers, first toast the buns. **(A)** Place a dollop of the mango chili sauce onto the bun, followed by **(B)** a mound of the red cabbage slaw. **(C)** Spoon some pan juices onto the chicken breasts, then place one onto the cabbage. Arrange 5 banana slices on top of the chicken. **(D)** Finally, place another scoop of mango chili sauce on top, followed by the toasted top bun. Done.

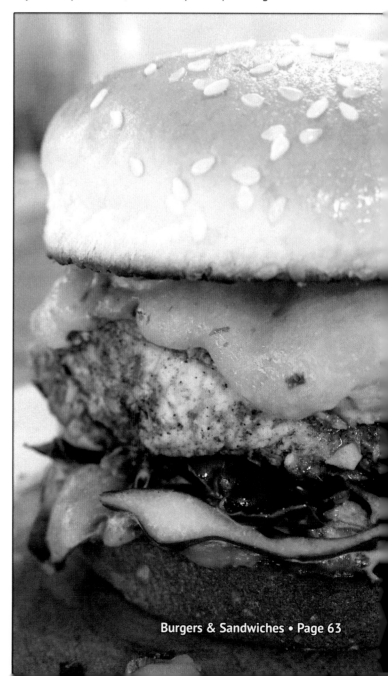

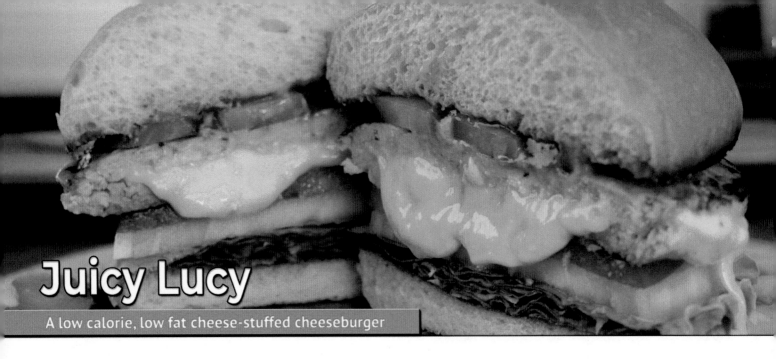

Juicy Lucy

A low calorie, low fat cheese-stuffed cheeseburger

To answer your question... no, I have absolutely no idea why this kind of burger is called a 'Juicy Lucy', but I can tell you that it's a simple and very tasty burger. It's pretty much a cheeseburger, where you stuff the cheese INSIDE of the patty, rather than melting it on top of the meat, like normal. Unlike most recipes, which call for stuffing enough full fat cheese into the burger, to choke a Wisconsinite... we're forming 2 thin ground turkey patties, then forming them together around a piece of low fat, low calorie, low point American or cheddar cheese.

Servings Info.:

Yields: 4 burgers
Servings: 4
Serving Size: 1 burger

Points:

	G	B	P
1 serving =	3	2	2
2 servings =	6	3	3
3 servings =	9	5	5
4 servings =	12	6	6

(These listed points DO NOT INCLUDE the bun. Use whichever brand buns or bread you want, then add these points. This is what's between the buns)

Ingredients:

Burger Patties :
- 1lb batch of my 'Savory' ground turkey mix, recipe in my "Cookbook Volume 1", on pg. 30. Form into 8 thin patties.
- 4 slices of Velveeta Original cheese slices, or any other brand of low point, low calorie sliced cheese.

Additional Toppings:
- Lettuce, any preferred variety.
- Sliced Onions
- Sliced Tomatoes
- Dill pickle slices
- Traditional yellow mustard
- 1/2 batch of my low point ketchup, recipe on page 22 of my "Cookbook Volume 2". Or... use any low point ketchup that you want, but adjust your points.

Directions:

1. Mix together the batch of meat. Form into a large mound, then divide into 8 sections.

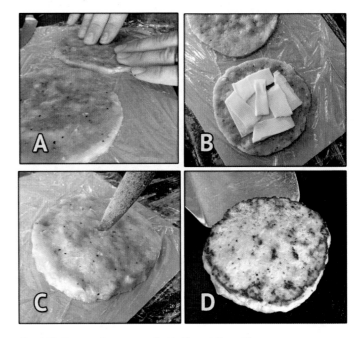

2. **(A)** Form the meat into 8 patties, then use your hands to make them more spread out/thin. **(B)** Break up a slice of cheese and lay it onto the center of 1 patty, leaving space around the edges. **(C)** Lay one patty over the first, sandwiching the cheese. Gently press on the sides to seal them, then poke a tiny hole into the top of the patty. **(D)** Preheat a large pan over medium heat for 1 minute. Spray with cooking spray, then cook the patties for 2 minutes per side.

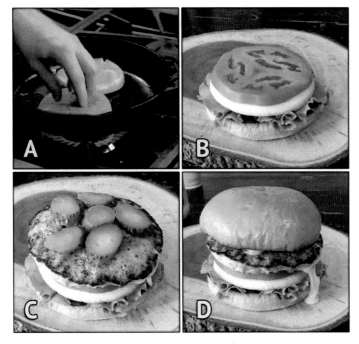

3. To assemble the burger, first **(A)** toast your buns... the burger buns, not your own. **(B)** Place some lettuce onto the bottom bun, followed by a slice of onion and then a slice of tomato. **(C)** Set the stuffed burger patty on top of the tomato, followed by a few dill pickle slices. **(D)** Smear the top bun with a little ketchup and mustard, then... go get a napkin. Done.

NOTES & SUGGESTIONS:

- *BURGER PATTIES:* Seriously... press them with your fingers, to spread them out and make them a little thinner and wider. Also, as pictured, leave a little space between the edges of the cheese and the edge of the meat.

- *CHEESE:* Though I used Velveeta Original slices for this recipe, you can use any low calorie/fat/point cheese that you want. In truth, the first burger should be 1 point lower than it shows. The recipe makes 4 burgers, so the points for ALL 4 burgers get added together, which is 6 points of cheese for all 4 burgers. If you only actually make 1 single burger, that 1 single burger's filling will only be 1 point on Blue/Purple, no change on Green. That's because one single slice of velveeta is only 1 point. You can use any brand or type of cheese you want. Ultra thin sliced provolone, Swiss... even smoked gouda and mozzarella. Go to the deli counter and ask them to slice you any cheese that you choose, AS THIN AS THEY CAN. Take it home, weigh a slice, in grams... and use a 1 or 2 point slice for your burger. I've tried this with smoked gouda, it's awesome. Also, 2 Tbsp of shredded part skim mozzarella is 1 point.

- *KETCHUP:* You don't have to make my recipe for ketchup. Use any low calorie/sugar/point brand of ketchup that you want. Adjust your points if necessary.

- *JUICY GIUSEPPE:* You could make a pretty gooey Italian version of this. Stuff it with mozzarella and hormel 70% reduced fat, turkey pepperoni. You can kick it up a notch by using my Italian sausage seasoning mix for the patty, instead of the 'savory'. Then you'd have a low point, fat and calorie stuffed pizza burger. Put some marinara sauce on top, instead of ketchup/mustard. Molto Bene!

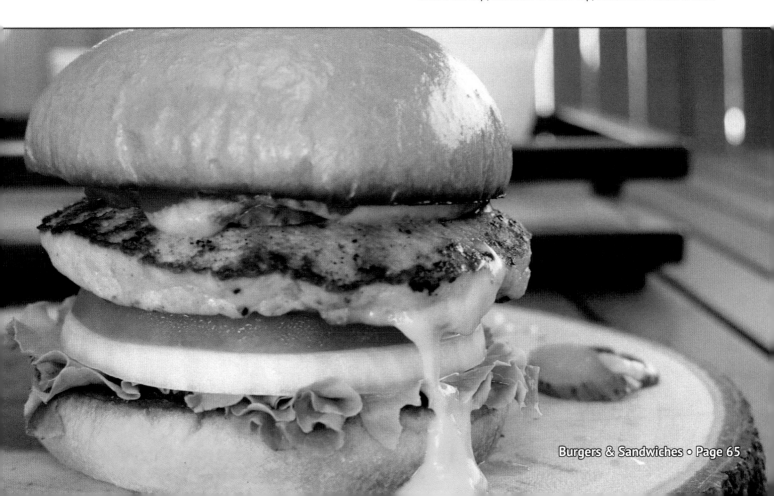

Lebanese Kafta

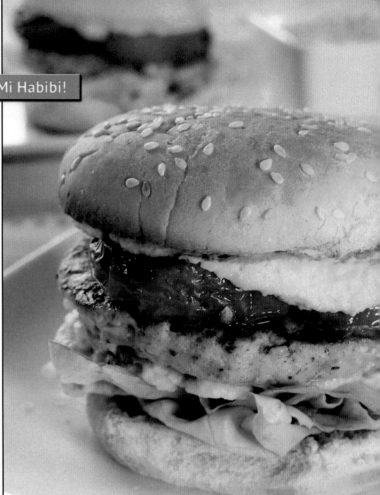

These Kafta burgers are my favorite of ALL of the ones that I've made so far. The flavors are just so freaking amazing, it'll blow your mind. We have an insanely delicious middle eastern spiced patty, sitting on a dollop of hummus, thin sliced red onion and lettuce. The patty is topped with thick slices of roasted roma tomato and is slathered with enough hummus to make a sultan sweat.

It's like going to a Kabab house and asking them to throw an entire shish kebab dinner onto a burger bun. If I was on death row and told I could only have one burger before being zapped... I'd pick this one, twice.

Servings Info.:

Yields: 4 burgers
Servings: 4
Serving Size: 1 burger

Points:

	G	B	P
1 serving =	2	1	1
2 servings =	5	1	1
3 servings =	7	2	2
4 servings =	9	2	2

(The GREEN, points assume that you greenies are using my "green-friendly" hummus recipe, from cookbook 2. ALSO: These listed points DO NOT INCLUDE the bun. Use whichever brand buns or bread you want, then add these points)

Ingredients:

Ground Turkey Kafta Patties
- 1/2 batch of my ground turkey "Kafta", recipe in my "Cookbook: Volume 1" on page 29. (Halve the recipe).
- Mix 1 Tablespoon of fat free plain greek yogurt into the raw meat mixture, for added moisture.

Low Point, Low Calorie Hummus
- 1 cup of my low calorie/low point Hummus, recipe in my "Cookbook: Volume 2" on page 21. Members on the Green plan are to use my "Green Friendly" hummus recipe.

Additional Vegetables:
- 1 medium red onion, thinly sliced across into thin rings
- Lettuce, whichever variety you prefer. I used butter lettuce.
- 4 good sized Roma tomatoes. Each roma tomato is to be sliced into thick slices, around 1/2 - 3/4 inch thick. 3 slices per burger.

Buns:
- 4 low point burger buns. I was able to find 3 point buns at my local store.

Directions:

1. First thing's first, the meat. Mix up a 1/2 batch of my ground turkey kafta, then cover it with plastic wrap and let it sit for 20 minutes. Once it's rested, move it to a cutting board and form into a ball. If the meat is a little tacky, lightly spray it with cooking spray to make it easier to manage.

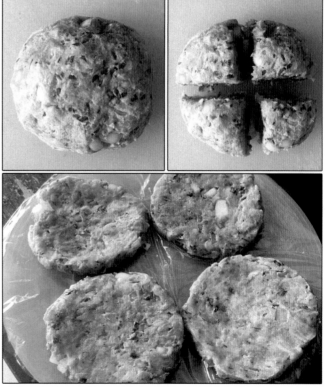

2. Slice the meat into 4 equal sections., then form each of the sections into patties. Set aside to allow the flavors to continue melding, as you prepare the rest of the ingredients.

3. Slice the red onion into thin slices, then set aside in a bowl. Wash off the lettuce and tear off a few good sized leaves. Pat them dry, with paper towels then set aside.

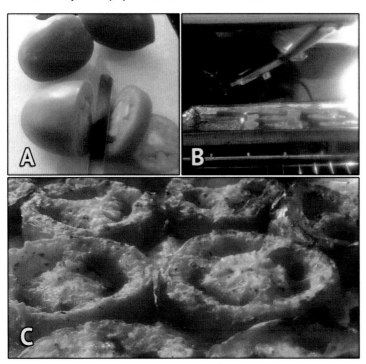

4. Preheat your oven to 425 degrees. Line a sheet pan with aluminum foil, then lightly spray with cooking spray. Turn on your oven's Broiler setting, to High, then prep the tomatoes. **(A)** Slice the Roma tomatoes into thick, 1/2" slices. Lay the tomatoes on the pan, spray with cooking spray and season with salt and black pepper on both sides. **(B)** Broil on the top rack for 6 minutes, rotate pan, then broil for another 5-6 minutes. **(C)** Remove from oven once the tomatoes are showing signs of charring... you want that. Set aside.

5. While the tomatoes are roasting, Heat a large pan over medium heat. Spray with cooking spray, then take your rested kafta patties and cook them until cooked through and browned on both sides. Remove from pan, set aside.

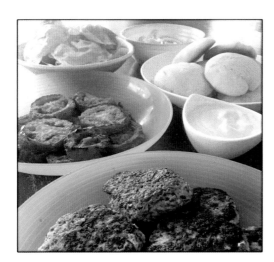

6. Now that you have all of the ingredients together, let's get to the best part, putting them together!

7. To assemble the burgers, first... toast your buns. Second, place some of the lettuce onto the bottom bun, then some red onion on top of the lettuce. Scoop 2 Tbsp of the low point hummus onto the red onions, then place a Kafta patty on top. Next, place 3 slices of the roasted tomatoes on top of the patty., then put 2 Tbsp of hummus on top of the tomatoes. Finally, cover with the top bun and enjoy. Belly dancing is optional, though it does give fit points.

NOTES & SUGGESTIONS:
- Yes, each burger has 1/4 cup of my hummus on it.
- I highly recommend using a decent amount of pepper on the tomatoes, it REALLY adds a great flavor when all the components are put together.
- Each burger patty measures in (raw) at around 3.5oz, because of the onions and parsley added into the meat.

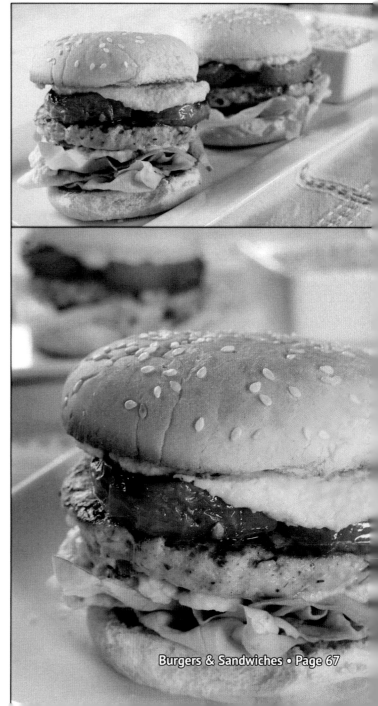

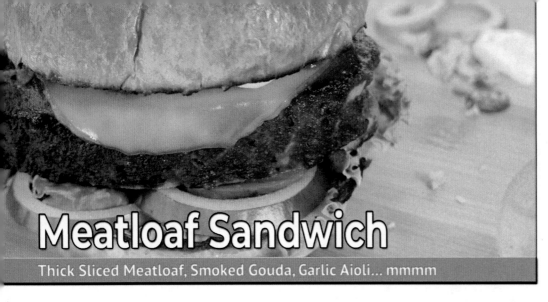

Meatloaf Sandwich

Thick Sliced Meatloaf, Smoked Gouda, Garlic Aioli... mmmm

Servings Info.:
Yields: 4 burgers
Servings: 4
Serving Size: 1 burger

Points:	G	B	P
1 serving =	5	3	3
2 servings =	10	6	6
3 servings =	14	9	9
4 servings =	19	12	12

Boy, talk about using every possible inch of paper on a page! Alright, this is my suped up, low fat version of Claim Jumper's meatloaf sandwich. I did my best to try and make a moist meatloaf using 99% fat free ground turkey and I'm pleased with the results. If you'd like it a tiiiiny bit fluffier, you can add a second egg white, because it won't affect the points for folks on the Green plan. But regardless, this is still a very tasty and filling sammich.

Ingredients:

Savory Ground Turkey Meatloaf Mix:
- 1lb batch of my Savory Ground Turkey, recipe in my "Cookbook: Volume 1", on page 30, with the following changes:
    - DO NOT USE THE BAKING SODA!!!!
    - Add 1 egg white
    - Add 2 Tbsp plain fat free Greek yogurt
    - Add 2 Tbsp CRUSHED rice krispies, to act as breadcrumbs
    - Do not include worcestershire sauce in the mix

Quick BBQ Sauce:
- 1 batch of my BBQ Sauce, recipe on pg. 14

Garlic Aioli Spread:
- 6 Tbsp plain fat free Greek yogurt
- 3-1/2 tsp light mayonnaise
- 2 tsp lemon juice
- 1/4 tsp garlic powder
- 2 medium cloves garlic, crushed, finely chopped
- 1/4 tsp salt
- 1/4 tsp pepper

Additional Ingredients:
- 3/4 cup diced onion, 1/2 cup diced celery, 1/4 cup diced carrot, 2 cloves garlic, minced. (set all of them aside).
- 4 slices smoked gouda, ultra thin sliced, around 12g each by weight. No more than 55g for the 4 slices.
- Thin sliced red onion
- Lettuce
- Dill pickle slices
- 4 Tbsp French's original french fried onions

Directions:

1 Bring all of the BBQ sauce ingredients to a simmer, in a small pot, for 2 minutes. Remove from heat, set aside.

2 Mix all of the garlic aioli ingredients together in a small cup. Cover and set aside.

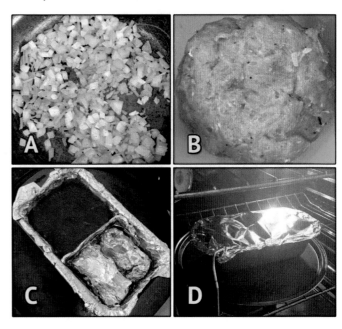

3 (A) Cook the diced onions, celery, carrots and garlic in a pan, with cooking spray. Season with salt and pepper, cook for 5-6 minutes, till vegetables are softened. Set aside.. (B) Mix together the 1lb batch of 'savory' meat seasoning, with the listed changes. Add in the cooked vegetables. The mix will be sticky, wet your hands, as needed, when mixing it (C) Pack the meat into one side of a 9" bread loaf pan and cover with some of the bbq sauce. Use foil to fill up the empty side of the pan, as pictured. (D) Heat oven to 375 degrees, then cover the pan with foil.

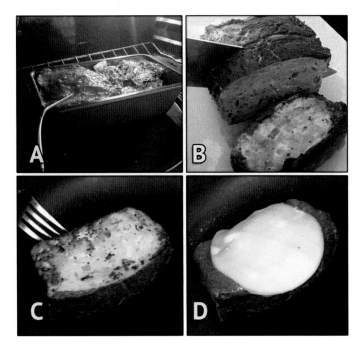

4 **(A)** Bake, covered at 375 degrees for 40 minutes, then remove the cover and bake 5 additional minutes. **(B)** Remove from oven and let sit for 15 minutes. Place the meatloaf on a cutting board and cut into 4 thick slices. **(C)** Heat a large pan over medium heat for 1 minute, then spray the slices with cooking spray and fry for 1 minute, then flip the slices. **(D)** Immediately spoon some bbq sauce onto each slice, then top with a thin slice of smoked gouda. Cover the pan and cook 1 more minute.

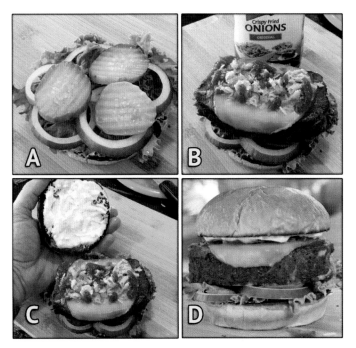

5 To assemble the sandwiches, first, toast your buns, then... **(A)** Place lettuce onto the bottom bun, followed by some red onion slices, then some pickles. **(B)** Place a slice of meatloaf on top of the pickles, then place a 1 Tbsp scoop of the fried onions onto the cheese. Drizzle a little bbq sauce over the top. **(C)** Smear a good scoop of the garlic aioli onto the top bun, then set it on top. **(D)** Done.

NOTES & SUGGESTIONS:

- *MEATLOAF MAYHEM:* Want to skip a whole heck of a lot of time and steps with this meatloaf? Skip making it in a loaf pan. You can just form all the meat, by hand, into a big meatloaf shape/mound, onto a baking pan. Smear it with BBQ sauce, loosely tent it with foil, and bake as directed. It won't look as pretty, but it'll definitely save on time. Plus... you won't use up half the foil in your house.
- *THIN SLICED SMOKED GOUDA???:* To get thin sliced smoked gouda, you'll need to go to your grocery store's deli department. Ask them to slice you some smoked gouda, AS THIN AS THEY CAN MAKE IT. When they sliced it for me, I took it home, weighed the slices, and they were each around 10 grams in weight, making the first slice 1 point, the 2nd slice 3 points, the 3rd slice 4 points and the 4th slice 6 points. The deli-guy said that the setting he used, was pretty much the universal "thinnest" setting they use at grocery stores. You can go up to 51 grams of smoked gouda for your 4 slices. Otherwise... adjust your points.
- *MEAT MIXTURE:* We had to remove the worcestershire sauce from the regular 'savory' meat recipe because that, combined with the worcestershire in the BBQ sauce, would have added an extra ingredient point.

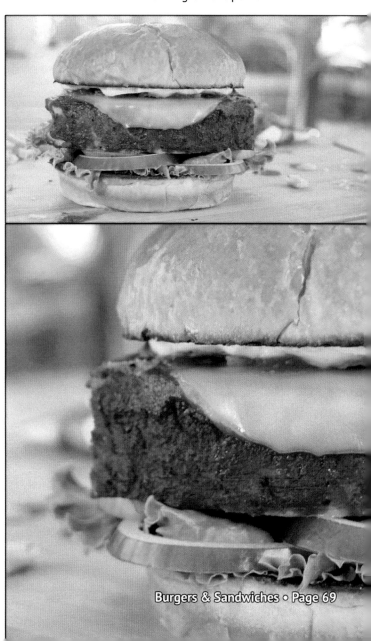

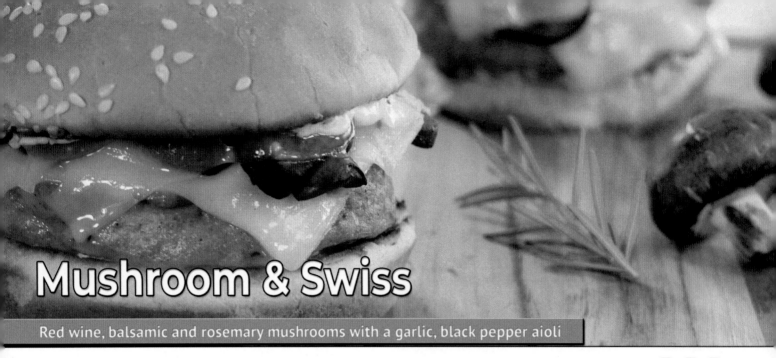

Mushroom & Swiss

Red wine, balsamic and rosemary mushrooms with a garlic, black pepper aioli

I've always liked a good mushroom burger, but the problem is that they're normally pretty high in points. I cut the calories, while amping the flavor, by cooking smarter. We're using 2 slices of deli thin sliced swiss cheese to hold the mushrooms in place. Speaking of mushrooms, these babies are cooked with red wine, beef broth, garlic and rosemary. Combining that with a deliciously creamy spread, kicks these up to healthy, yet gourmet.

Servings Info.:

Yields: 4 burgers
Servings: 4
Serving Size: 1 burger

Points:

	G	B	P
1 serving =	5	3	3
2 servings =	11	6	6
3 servings =	16	9	9
4 servings =	21	12	12

*(These listed points **DO NOT INCLUDE** the bun. Use whichever brand buns or bread you want, then add these points. These listed points are also for 1/4lb patties.)*

Ingredients:

Savory Ground Turkey Patties:
- 1lb batch of my "Savory" ground turkey recipe, in my "Cookbook: Volume 1", on page 30**

Black Pepper & Garlic Aioli Spread:
- 1/2 cup fat free plain Greek yogurt
- 1 Tbsp light/reduced fat mayonnaise
- 1 tsp lemon juice
- 2 medium garlic cloves, crushed and minced.
- 1/4 tsp black pepper
- 1/4 tsp garlic powder
- pinch of salt, to taste
- 1 tsp reduced fat parmesan grated topping, like Kraft brand**

Mushrooms:
- 2 (8oz) packages of sliced baby bella (cremini) mushrooms
- 1 medium garlic clove, minced
- 1/4 cup fat free beef broth
- 1 Tbsp red wine
- 2 tsp balsamic vinegar
- 1/4 tsp pepper
- 1/4 tsp salt
- 1 tsp fresh rosemary, finely chopped

• Additional Ingredients:
8 slices ultra thin sliced swiss cheese, such as Sargento or Jarslberg brand. (11 total points)**

Directions:

1. Combine all of the Aioli ingredients in a small bowl. Stir to combine, cover and set aside in the fridge, so the flavors can meld together.

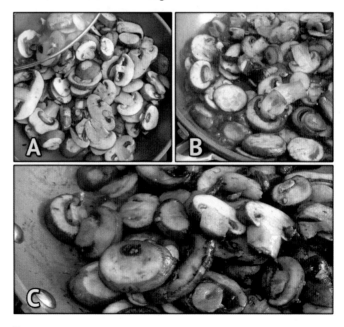

2. **(A)** Using cooking spray, cook the mushrooms and garlic in a large sauce pan, covered, for 5 minutes. **(B)** Add the beef broth, red wine, vinegar, salt, pepper and rosemary. **(C)** Cook, uncovered, over medium heat for 8 to 10 minutes, or until most all of the liquid has evaporated. Turn off heat, cover the pan, set aside.

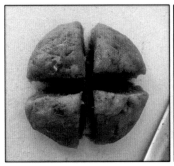
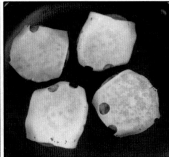

3. For this recipe, we're making larger 1/4lb patties. Divide your batch of prepared meat into 4 sections, then form into patties and cook on both sides. Melt 1 slice of the thin swiss cheese on top of each patty.

4. To assemble the burgers, toast the buns, then **(A)** spread 1 Tbsp of the aioli onto each bun. **(B)** Place a turkey patty onto the bottom bun, followed by a mound of mushrooms. **(C)** Place the 2nd slice of cheese on top of the hot mushrooms (rewarm them if they cooled off), then finish with the top bun. **(D)** Done.

NOTES & SUGGESTIONS:

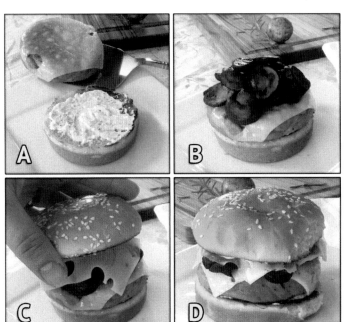

- **POINTS:** This is primarily for folks on GREEN. In this recipe, I am using a thicker 1/4 lb patty, which is 2 points for you guys, because other than mushrooms, there isn't much on this burger. If you want your burger to be 1 point lower, make a thinner 2oz patty and your first burger will drop to 4 points. Add some produce or 0 point filler to build up the burger, if you go with the thinner patty.
- **CHEESE:** 2 slices of thin sliced sargento brand swiss cheese are 3 points. NORMAL thickness swiss cheese is usually 3 points. So, it gives you options. You can use 2 thin slices, like I did, which are used to keep the 'shrooms from falling out of your burger when you bite it. Or, you can use 1 regular, thicker, 3 point slice on the patty, it's your call. There are 11 total points of swiss cheese for these 4 burgers, as is.
- **THIN SLICED CHEESE:** If you can't find sargento or a different brand "thin" sliced swiss cheese, go to your store's deli section and ask them to cut the cheese for you. Yes... I went there. When you tell them to cut the cheese... tell them you want VERY thin slices, not regular thickness.
- **MUSHROOMS:** Use any variety of mushroom you want. You can also use additional mushrooms, chopped up and mixed into the meat, to add more bulk and savoriness to the patties.

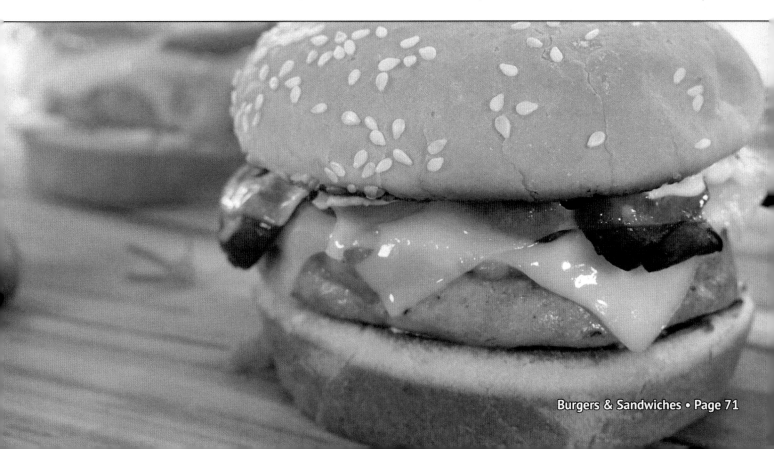

Oktoberfest

Grab your Lederhosen, we're headed to Deutschland!

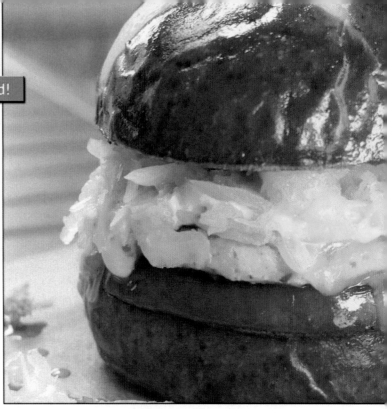

Who says that Oktoberfest only comes around once per year?! This baby's got enough German cred to give David Hasselhoff a run for his money. I'm pulling out all the cliches I can think of, to pack a blitzkrieg of flavor into this bad boy.

Though you can use any buns you want, this burger is so low in points that I opted for a high point pretzel bun for my pictures, but... use any type that you would like.

This culinary Hans & Franz is loaded with a pan seared, thick slice of red onion and a low point bratwust patty, topped with swiss cheese, a mustard-beer sauce and a pile of sauerkraut. Did I mention... 0 point mustard-beer sauce!?!?!

Servings Info.:
Yields: 4 burgers
Servings: 4
Serving Size: 1 burger

Points:

	G	B	P
1 serving =	2	1	1
2 servings =	5	3	3
3 servings =	7	4	4
4 servings =	10	6	6

*(These listed points **DO NOT INCLUDE** the bun. Use whichever brand buns or bread you want, then add these points. These listed points are for a 2-3oz patty, for Greenies.)*

Ingredients:

Low Point Bratwurst Patties:
• 1/2 pound batch of my low point Bratwurst, sectioned into 4 thin patties. Recipe in my "Cookbook: Volume 1", pg. 26.

Mustard Beer Sauce: *(Makes 1/2 cup, 0 total points)*
• 2 Tbsp (1oz) Light Beer. Yes.... light beer, deal with it.
• 1 Tbsp dijon mustard
• 2 Tbsp traditional yellow mustard
• 1 Tbsp whole grain, stone ground mustard
• 2 Tbsp fat free plain Greek yogurt
• 1/2 tsp dry mustard powder
• 1/4 tsp salt
• 1/4 tsp pepper
• a dash of hot sauce, to taste (optional)

Additional Ingredients:
• 4 thick slices of red onion, around 1/2 inch thick.
• Sauerkraut. It can be found by the refrigerated pickles at the grocery store.
• 4 slices Swiss cheese. Reduced fat, or thin sliced, such as Sargento brand thin sliced Swiss. *(see notes)****
• 4 Cornichon/Gherkin, fancy lil French pickles. (optional)

Directions:

1. Mix the 1/2lb batch of Bratwurst, as directed in Cookbook 1 and set aside. After 20 minutes, form into 4 patties. If the mixture is tacky, wet your hands while forming the meat.

2. Mix together all of the ingredients for the Mustard Beer sauce, till smooth. Cover and set aside.

3. Toast your buns (BURGER BUNS, sicko!), then set aside.

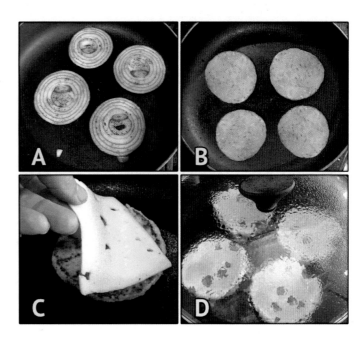

4. **(A)** Heat a large pan over medium heat for 1 minute, or until water sizzles off its surface. Spray the onion slices with cooking spray, season with salt and pepper, then place into the pan. Cook for 2 minutes per side, then set aside. **(B)** In the same pan, cook the Bratwurst patties with cooking spray. Cook for 2 minutes over medium heat, then **(C)** flip the burgers and top with Swiss cheese slices. **(D)** Cover pan with a lid, cook for 2 additional minutes, then remove patties from pan and set aside.

5. To assemble the sandwiches, **(A)** place one of the red onion slices onto the bottom bun, **(B)** followed by one of the bratwurst patties. Spoon 1 Tbsp of mustard sauce onto the swiss cheese. **(C)** Take a good scoop of the Sauerkraut from the jar and give it a little squeeze, to remove some of the vinegar brine. Place the Kraut on top of the sauce. It should resemble the top of Guy Fieri's head at this point. **(D)** Lastly, smear 1 more Tablespoon of mustard sauce onto the top bun, then set it on top of the sauerkraut. If you want… you can skewer a small Gherkin pickle with a toothpick, then top your burger with it. Man… the French just can't win.

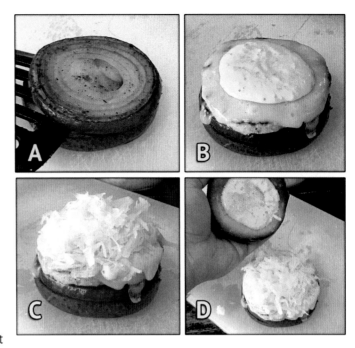

NOTES & SUGGESTIONS:

- *CHEESE:* 2 slices of Sargento brand thin sliced swiss cheese are 3 points. NORMAL thickness swiss cheese is usually 3 points. So, it gives you options. You can use 1 thin slice per burger, like I did, which makes the points for the cheese 1 point on the first burger, 3 for the second, 4 for the 3rd and 6 for the 4th serving of cheese. Or, you can simply scan different brands of Swiss cheese, use whatever you want, and adjust the points of the recipe. Either way… it's a low point burger.
- *THIN SLICED CHEESE:* If you can't find sargento or a different brand "thin" sliced swiss cheese, go to your store's deli section and ask them to cut the cheese for you. Yes… I went there. When you tell them to cut the cheese… tell them you want VERY thin slices, not regular thickness.
- *MUSTARD BEER SAUCE/SPREAD:* If you don't want to use alcohol for your spread, then use water, it still tastes great.
- *SAUERKRAUT:* This is honestly the first time in my life I've tried it. If you don't mind eating pickles or pickled vegetables, you'll like it.
- *GHERKIN PICKLES:* I wasn't planning to putting fancy French pickles on top of the burger, as garnish. However, as soon as I pulled the Bratwurst out of the fridge, the pickles surrendered. Luckily, the Swiss acted as a neutral buffer between the two.
- *3 MUSTARDS???*: Over 1 Tbsp of whole grain mustard is 1 point. Over 1 Tbsp of dijon mustard is a point. But, if we add both of them together, you now have 2 Tbsp of mustard, that stays 0 points in the recipe builder. By using loopholes like this, we are able to combine different types of mustard, to make 1/2 cup of 0 point mustard spread.

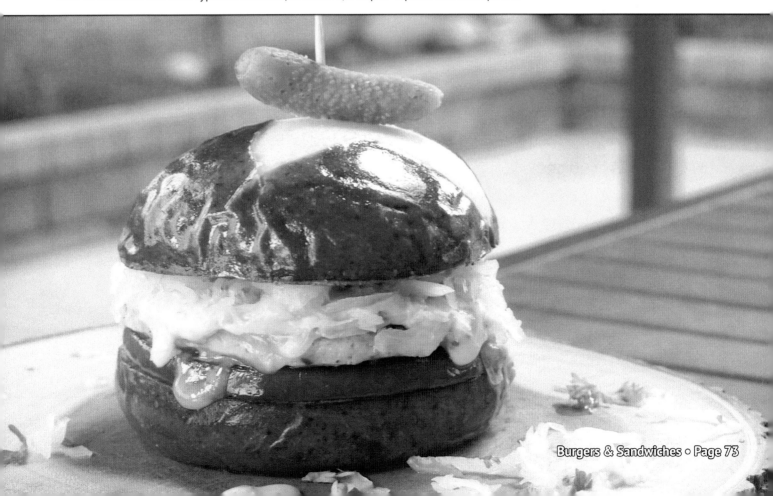

Orange Chicken

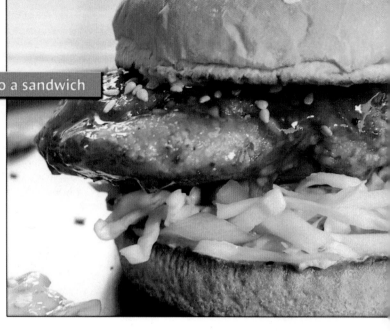

My favorite pre-WW junk food was the Orange Chicken from Panda Express. I haven't had it in ages, because of how high it is in points and calories. When I was thinking of unique and snazzy chicken sandwich ideas for the final few entries of this section, it hit me like a roundhouse kick from Kung Fu panda... "Why don't I make a Panda Express-ish sandwich?" I took inspiration from an incredibly high point recipe I found online, then I hacked the heck out of it with the recipe builder. The sauce for this sandwich is actually a combination of 2 sauces: Panda's Orange Chicken and the sauce used for General Tso's chicken. So... as you can imagine, the flavor in this sauce has tremeeeeeendous depth.

Ingredients:

Breaded Chicken Breasts:
- 4 (4oz) Boneless, skinless chicken breasts. The 4 oz limit is for Greenies.
- Breading: Prepare 1 batch of my "breading 2.0", recipe in my "Cookbook: Volume 1", on page 35. Remember, if you're on the Green plan, use egg whites, not the whole eggs.

Asian Green Cabbage & Scallion Slaw:
- 1/2 head of green cabbage, sliced very thin.
- 1/4 cup green onion sliced thin, at an angle. Use both the green and white parts (takes about 4 whole green onions).
- 1 Tbsp rice wine vinegar (in the Asian food aisle).
- 2 Tbsp lemon juice
- 1/4 tsp sesame oil
- 2 tsp 0 point sweetener o' choice
- 1/4 tsp salt
- 1/4 tsp pepper

Asian Chili Aioli:
- 2-1/2 Tbsp fat free plain Greek yogurt
- 1 tsp light mayonnaise
- 1 to 2 tsp Asian chili sauce
- 1/4 tsp pepper
- 1 tsp lemon juice
- 1 tsp low sodium soy sauce

AWESOME Orange Sauce/Glaze:
- 1/4 cup orange juice
- 1 Tbsp orange peel, finely chopped
- 3 Tbsp reduced sodium soy sauce
- 4 Tbsp 0 point sweetener o' choice
- 2 medium garlic cloves, minced
- 1 tsp ginger root, finely chopped/minced
- 1/8 tsp red pepper flakes
- 1-1/2 tsp cornstarch, dissolved in 2 Tbsp water.
- 1 Tbsp sugar free syrup (pancake syrup)
- *** 1 tsp sesame seeds, toasted, for garnish.

Servings Info.:
Yields: 4 sandwiches
Servings: 4
Serving Size: 1 sandwich

Points:

	G	B	P
1 serving =	2	1	1
2 servings =	5	3	3
3 servings =	7	4	4
4 servings =	9	5	5

(These listed points DO NOT INCLUDE the bun. Use whichever brand buns or bread you want, then add these points. This is what's between the buns)

Directions:

1. Mix the cabbage and slaw ingredients together, set aside. Mix the asian chili aioli ingredients together, set aside.

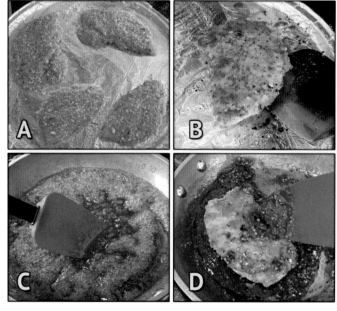

2. Preheat oven to 425 degrees. **(A)** Bread the chicken, spray with cooking spray and bake for 14 minutes. **(B)** Flip and cook for 8 more minutes. **(C)** Heat all of the orange sauce ingredients (minus the sesame seeds) in a pan. Bring to a rolling boil for 2-3 minutes, till thick. **(D)** Coat the chicken breasts in sauce, turn off heat.

3. To toast the sesame seeds, heat them in a small pan over medium heat till lightly browned and fragrant. It'll take 3-4 minutes. Instructions can be found in my "Cookbook: Volume 1", on page 47.

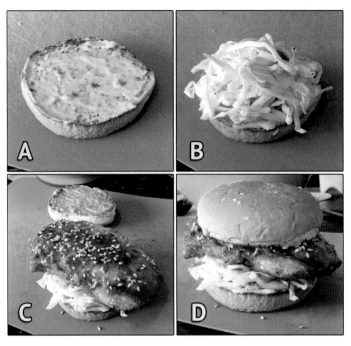

4. **(A)** Toast your sandwich buns or bread o' choice, then place dollop of the Asian chili aioli on the bottom bun. **(B)** Set a small mound of the green cabbage slaw on top, **(C)** followed by one of the glazed chicken breasts. Sprinkle 1/4 tsp of the toasted sesame seeds on top of the chicken and spread some more of the aioli onto the top bun. **(D)** Place the bun on top, get your grub on.

NOTES & SUGGESTIONS:

- *CHICKEN:* Blue & Purple folks can use Dolly Parton sized chicken breasts. However, you Green folks should use chicken that is an appropriate size (in ounces) to not go above 1 point per sandwich.
- *GREEN CABBAGE 'SLAW:* A couple of things:
  *Obviously, remove the hard core from the bottom of the cabbage.
  * Slice the cabbage very thin, if you don't, it'll be hard to place into a nice mound on the bun.
  * Use regular sugar if you want, but adjust your points.
- *BREADING:* My Rice Krispies breading recipe is lower in points and calories than an equal amount of regular breading. However, you Gluten Free folks, please make note that KELLOGG'S brand Rice Krispies is not Gluten Free. Make sure to find a gluten free brand, or use another cereal that is low points for 1-1/4 cups, such as rice chex.
- *CHILI SAUCE:* In the Asian food aisle, by the soy sauce, you'll find the chili sauces. I used the "Huy Fong Foods" brand chili garlic sauce. They're the folks that make Sriracha sauce. Most major grocery stores carry it.
- *ORANGE SAUCE:* This sauce is freakin' bomb.com awesome. If you are allergic to sweeteners, you can use regular sugar instead of sweetener (I used lakonta monkfruit). The points increase can be reduced by using reduced sugar orange juice, to offset the extra points from regular sugar.
  * Here's a great idea. You can use my breading recipe to slice up, bread, then bake, around 18-24 chunks of chicken breast. That'll give you a pile of breaded and baked crispy nuggets for 4 points (not counting the points for chicken, on Green). You can THEN toss all of that chicken with a batch of this sauce and garnish with the sesame seeds. Congrats... you have a platter of delicious, low fat, low calorie Orange Chicken.

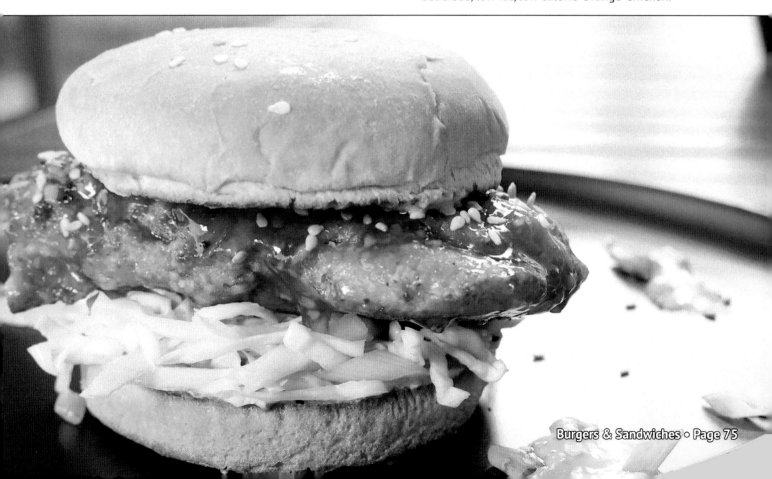

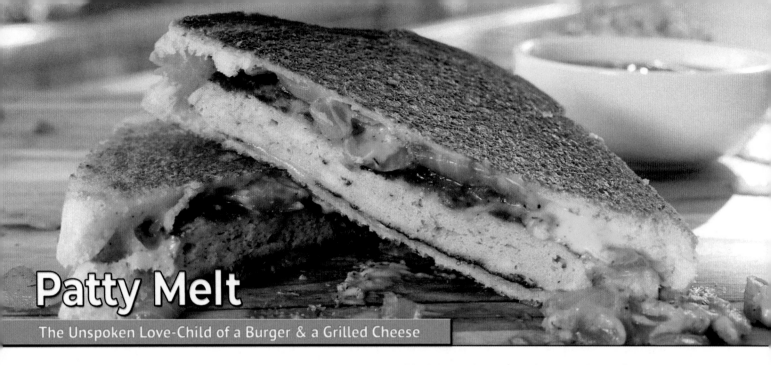

Patty Melt

The Unspoken Love-Child of a Burger & a Grilled Cheese

Ever wondered what'd happen, if a burger hooked up with a grilled cheese it met at a bar one night, after one too many jello shots? Well, 9 months later, you'd see a baby Patty Melt on a "Who's the daddy?" episode of Maury. When that happens, you get a burger patty topped with caramelized onions, in the middle of a grilled cheese sandwich.... with serious daddy issues.

Servings Info.:
Yields: 4 sandwiches
Servings: 4
Serving Size: 1 sandwich

Points:

	G	B	P
1 serving =	5	3	3
2 servings =	9	6	6
3 servings =	14	9	9
4 servings =	18	12	12

(These listed points DO NOT INCLUDE the bun. Use whichever brand buns or bread you want, then add these points. This is what's between the buns)

Ingredients:

Ground Turkey Pattys:
• 1/2 lb batch of my Savory Ground Turkey, recipe in my "Cookbook: Volume 1", on page 30.

'Beefy' Caramelized Onions:
• 2 large onions, diced
• 0 point cooking spray
• 1 medium garlic clove, chopped
• 1/2 cup beef broth, fat free
• 1/2 tsp salt
• 1/4 tsp black pepper (use white pepper if'ya want)
• 1/2 tsp onion powder

Additional Ingredients:
• 8 slices of low point cheese. For THIS recipe, I am using 4 slices of Velveeta Original singles and 4 slices of Sargento ultra thin sliced colby/jack. *(SEE NOTES)****
• Butter flavored cooking spray *(SEE NOTES)****
• 8 slices of low point bread (I am not including the bread in the points for this recipe, which is my norm... *(SEE NOTES)****

Directions:

1. Mix the 1/2 batch of 'savory' ground turkey meat, then form it into 4 patties. Set aside to rest for 20 minutes.

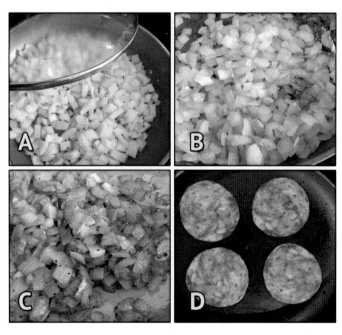

2. (A) Use cooking spray to cook the onions and garlic, covered, for 10 minutes on medium heat. Stir occasionally, so they don't burn. **(B)** Remove the lid after 10 minutes, then add the beef broth, salt, pepper and onion powder. **(C)** Reduce heat to medium-low and simmer for 6-8 minutes, or until all of the liquid has evaporated. Set aside. **(D)** Preheat a large pan for 1 minute over medium heat. Spray with cooking spray and cook the burger patties for 2 minutes per side. Set aside.

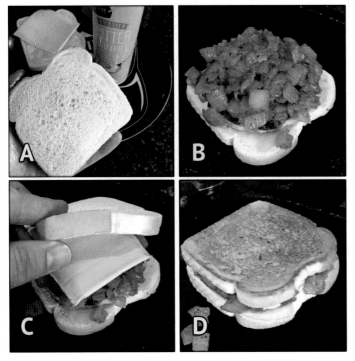

NOTES & SUGGESTIONS:

- **CHEESE:** Ok, these notes are going to have a loooot of info. The big reason is the cheese. THIS is where you can customize the heck out of this sandwich. You are aiming to use 2 slices of cheese that will be no more than 3 points total. You can use 2 slices of velveeta originals, which is 3 points... or you can use 1 slice of velveeta and 1 slice of sargento ultra thin sliced colby jack, like I did. Try scanning different brands of "ultra thin" sliced deli cheeses. You can also ask your local deli to slice you any cheese you want, AS THIN AS POSSIBLE. When you get home, weigh the slices in grams, with your kitchen scale. In this recipe, there are 12 points of cheese for all 8 slices.

- **BREAD:** The bread that I used "natures own: butter bread" is 3 points for 2 slices. There are brands that are 1 point PER slice, such as Sara Lee 45 calorie bread, my store has it, but only the whole wheat variety... I prefer white bread with my patty melts. If you end up using bread that is more or less points than 3 points for 2 slices... adjust your points per serving.

- **BUTTER 'FLAVORED' COOKING SPRAY:** Not all brands of cooking spray are 'true' 0 point sprays. There are some that only let you use 4-8 seconds of spray before it adds points. I have found that the generic store brands, such as 'great value' at walmart and the 'signature select' brands at albertsons, vons, ralphs and krogers... stay 0 points in the app, even if you use them to paint a Buick. Scan your cooking spray and make sure to use a 0 point amount on each sandwich. In my case, I do a good 2 second burst from about 6 inches away, to ensure that each bread slice gets a nice coating. I only use the brands that stay 0 points in the recipe builder. Use what you like, but adjust points. You can also spread Greek yogurt onto your bread, like you would butter... to get a nice crust. However, the extra Greek yogurt will add a point, for folks on the Green plan.

- **WHERE'S THE RYE or SOURDOUGH?:** Nobody makes low point rye bread. You can always add caraway seeds to the onions. For sourdough, 'Healthy Life' makes a 35 calorie per slice, sourdough. Check your local stores.

3. **(A)** Use butter flavored cooking spray, to spray 1 side of each piece of bread with a good 1 second burst. Then heat the same pan that you cooked the burgers in for a minute, over medium-low heat. **(B)** Place 1 slice of bread (for each sandwich) 'butter' side down on the pan. Place 1 slice of cheese on the bread, followed by your burger patty, then put a good sized mound of your caramelized onions on top of the patty. **(C)** Place another slice of cheese on top of the onions, followed be the 2nd piece of bread. Spray the top of the bread with cooking spray. **(D)** Cook the sandwich over medium-low heat for a few minutes, until it is brown and toasted on the bottom. Then flip your sandwich and toast the other side. Keep an eye on it, so it doesn't burn.

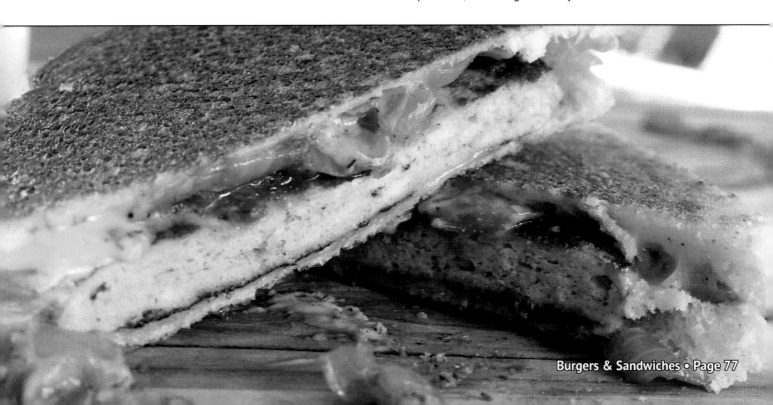

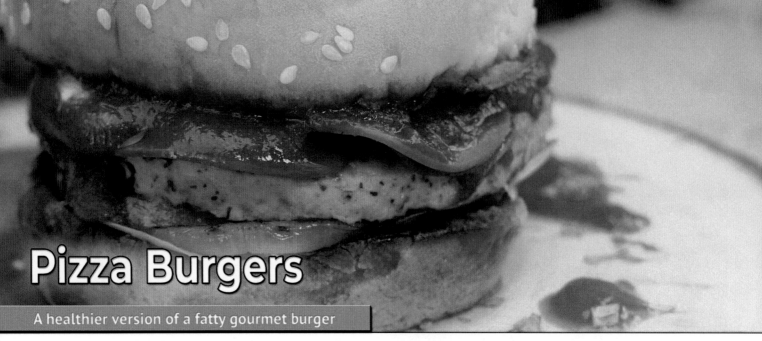

Pizza Burgers

A healthier version of a fatty gourmet burger

I recently watched a show on the food network that had a pizza burger. Of course, it had enough grease, fat and calories to make you gain 5lbs just looking at it.

My version has a roasted garlic spread, fresh basil, charred onion, an Italian sausage patty, mozzarella, pepperoni and marinara sauce. I've included directions in the notes for a "Supreme" pizza version.

Servings Info.:
Yields: 4 burgers
Servings: 4
Serving Size: 1 burger

Points:

	G	B	P
1 serving =	3	2	2
2 servings =	6	4	4
3 servings =	9	6	6
4 servings =	12	8	8

(These listed points DO NOT INCLUDE the bun. Use whichever brand buns or bread you want, then add these points.)

Ingredients:

Savory Ground Turkey Patties
- 1/2 batch of my "Italian Sausage" ground turkey recipe, in my "Cookbook: Volume 1" on page 28, with the following changes:
  - *Toast the fennel seeds, as shown in Cookbook 1, on pg. 47.*

Roasted Garlic Spread
- 16-20 garlic cloves, preferably still in their skin.
- Tin foil
- Cooking spray
- 2 tsp water (trust me)

Marinara Sauce
- You can use ANY 0 point marinara sauce you want, or... use my fast and easy "5 Minute Marinara" recipe, recipe on page 14.

Additional Ingredients:
- 6 Tbsp part-skim, shredded mozzarella cheese. Scan it, make sure what you buy is 4 points for 6 Tbsp..
- 32 pieces Hormel 70% less fat turkey pepperoni (4 points)
- 1 large onion, sliced into (4) 1/2 inch thick rounds.
- Fresh basil leaves

Directions:

1. Mix together the ground meat, set aside for 20 minutes. Form the meat into 4 patties, cover, then set aside.

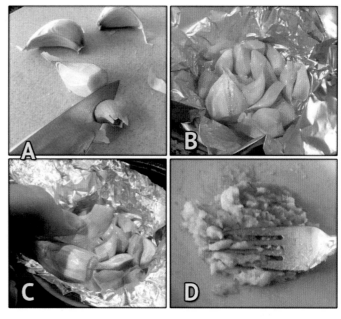

2. Preheat oven to 375 degrees. **(A)** Slice the ends off of 16-20 fresh cloves of garlic, still in the skin. **(B)** Place all of the garlic into a pouch made of tin foil, then spray with cooking spray. Close the foil pouch and bake at 375 degrees for 45 minutes. **(C)** Remove from oven, then pick up each garlic clove and gently squeeze the back end, which will cause the roasted garlic to fall out. Place all garlic cloves into a dish. **(D)** Add the water to the garlic cloves, then mash with a fork till smooth. Seal in an air tight container and set aside.

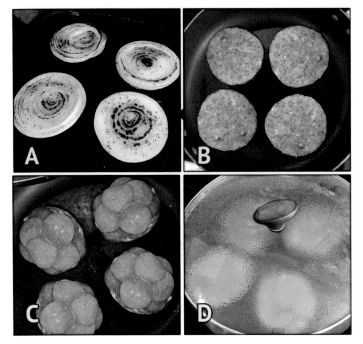

- *Marinara:* Use whatever brand you want, make your own, or make mine, as long as it's a 0 point sauce.
- *Roasted Garlic:* There are different ways you can prepare garlic for roasting. You can slice across an entire bulb of garlic, like you see on cooking shows. I chose not to show that method, so that less experienced cooks wouldn't risk losing a limb. You can cut individual cloves like I did, cut through an entire head, as is typical, or use my slow cooker roasted garlic recipe. Any way works. There IS no wrong way, it's all personal preference.
- I have toasting the fennel seeds, as an optional step... but sweet baby Jesus, I swear to you that it makes suuuuuuuch a huge flavor difference in the meat.
- *CHEESE:* Use any cheese you want, whether shredded or sliced, thin sliced provolone or mozzarella. As long as you keep it to 1 point per burger. Otherwise, adjust the points.
- *SUPREME PIZZA VERSION:* To make a Supreme version, top this baby like you would a pizza. Add some cooked green bell peppers, sauteed mushrooms, black olives... make it your own! Heck, if you want to ignite a furious battle for the ages, add Canadian bacon and pineapple for a Hawaiian burger! *evil cackle*

3. **(A)** Heat a pan over medium heat for a minute, spray with cooking spray, then cook the 4 sliced onion rounds for 2 minutes per side, seasoning with salt and pepper. Set aside. **(B)** In the same pan, cook the sausage patties for 2 minutes on medium heat. **(C)** Flip the patties, then quickly place 1-1/2 Tbsp mozzarella onto each patty, then place 8 slices of "light" pepperoni onto each burger. **(D)** Cover with a lid and cook for another 1-1/2 minutes. Remove patties from the pan and start building your burgers, Paisanos!

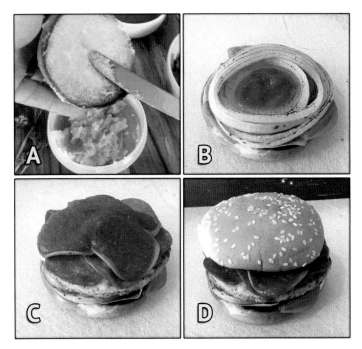

4. To assemble the burgers, first toast the buns, then **(A)** spread some of the roasted garlic onto each bun. **(B)** Place a few leaves of fresh basil onto the bottom bun, followed by one of the charred onion rounds and a dollop of marinara sauce. **(C)** Place the sausage patty (with mozzarella and pepperoni) on top of the onion slice, and cover with a scoop of marinara sauce. **(D)** Finally, cover with the top bun that has been smeared with roasted garlic.

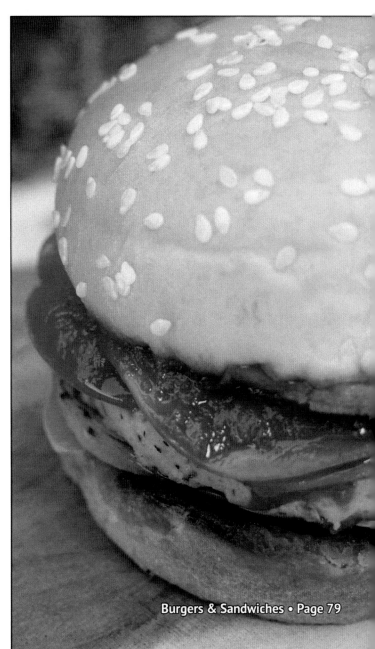

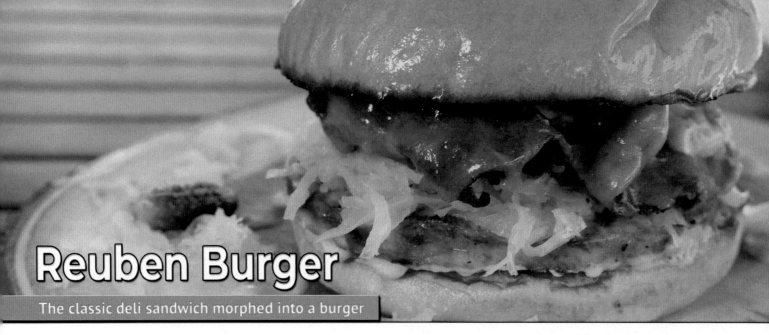

Reuben Burger

The classic deli sandwich morphed into a burger

When you think of a classic deli sandwich, from one of those little mom and pop deli's, there are 3 that immediately come to mind for most people: corned beef, pastrami on rye and a reuben. A reuben is a pastrami sandwich's tough older brother that's spent time in the joint and has some attitude. A typical reuben sandwich has thousand island dressing, sauerkraut and a thick pile of pastrami with melted swiss cheese. To make this low point burger version, we're using deli thin cut pastrami, so we can get a good amount for only 1 point added onto each burger. Then, we're using thin sliced swiss cheese, my thousand island salad dressing and placing it on one of my low point 'savory' ground turkey patties.

Servings Info.:
Yields: 4 burgers
Servings: 4
Serving Size: 1 burger

Points: (G) (B) (P)

	G	B	P
1 serving =	4	2	2
2 servings =	7	4	4
3 servings =	9	7	7
4 servings =	12	9	9

(These listed points DO NOT INCLUDE the bun. Use whichever brand buns or bread you want, then add these points. This is what's between the buns)

Ingredients:

Burger Patties:
- 1/2 batch of my "savory" ground turkey mix, formed into 4 patties. Recipe in my "Cookbook: Volume 1" on pg. 30.

Thousand Island Dressing:
- 1 batch of my low point thousand island dressing. Recipe on pg. 21.

Additional Toppings:
- Sauerkraut. You can find it in the grocery store, near the jarred pickles.
- 4 slices Swiss cheese, thin sliced. *(see notes)***
- Thin cut pastrami, up to 4 points worth, divided into four portions. *(SEE NOTES!!)***

Directions:

1. Prepare a 1/2 batch of my thousand island dressing. Cover and set aside.

2. Preheat a pan over medium heat for 1 minute. Spray with cooking spray and cook the patties for 2 minutes per side. Remove and set aside.

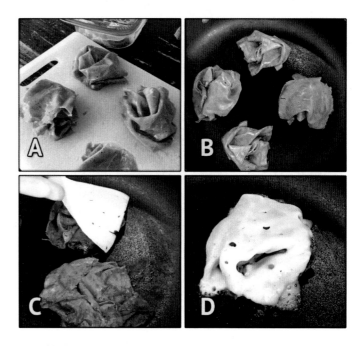

3. **(A)** Separate your thin cut pastrami into four 1 point mounds. **(B)** Sear the 4 pastrami mounds in a hot pan, over medium heat, for 1 minute. **(C)** Flip the pastrami and cover with a Swiss cheese slice. **(D)** Cook for 1 more minute, then remove from heat.

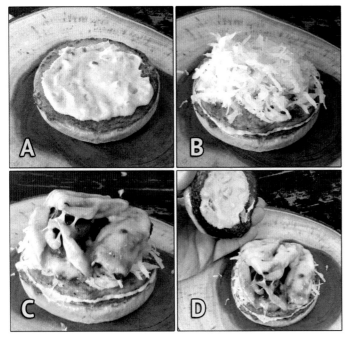

4. **(A)** Toast your sandwich buns o' choice, then smear the bottom bun with a scoop of thousand island dressing. **(B)** Place a burger patty on the dressing, then squeeze the juice from a fist full of sauerkraut and place it on top. **(C)** Next, set one of the mounds of hot pastrami and melted swiss onto the 'kraut. **(D)** Finally, smear some more thousand island onto the top bun. Done.

NOTES & SUGGESTIONS:

- **DRESSING:** Don't like thousand island? Use deli mustard, just make sure to use a 0 point amount. Some brands of deli style stone ground mustard allow you to use 1 Tbsp for 0 points, some only let you use 2 tsp. Scan your brand. What I normally do as a trick, for more 0 point mustard... I'll mix a 0 point amount of whole grain/stone ground mustard with 1 Tbsp of dijon mustard. It'll stay 0 points in the builder.
- **Sauerkraut:** If you don't like the thought of a big pile of pickled cabbage on your burger, replace it with lettuce and tomato, so that you can have a regular pastrami burger.
- **Pastrami:** I found "hillshire farms, deli thin cut pastrami" at the grocery store, in the cold cut meat section. A 7oz package is ONLY 4 points!!! For all of it! There were 13 large slices in the container. I divided it into 4 portions, so each burger got 3 slices for 1 point... don't ask what happened to the extra slice. *cough*
  Use any brand of thin cut pastrami, or thin cut turkey pastrami you want. You can even go to the deli counter and ask them to slice you some pastrami as thin as they can. Then go home and measure the meat by weight, in grams. Use a 1 point amount, per burger.
- **Swiss Cheese:** 2 slices of Sargento brand thin sliced swiss cheese are 3 points. NORMAL thickness swiss cheese is usually 3 points. So, it gives you options. You can use 1 thin slice per sandwich, like I did, which makes the points for the cheese 1 point on the first burger, 3 for the second, 4 for the 3rd and 6 for the 4th serving of cheese. Or, you can simply scan different brands of Swiss cheese, use whatever you want, and adjust the points of the recipe. Also, you can ask the folks at the deli counter to slice you some Swiss cheese, as thin as they possibly can. Then when you get home, weigh it, in grams, to check the points.

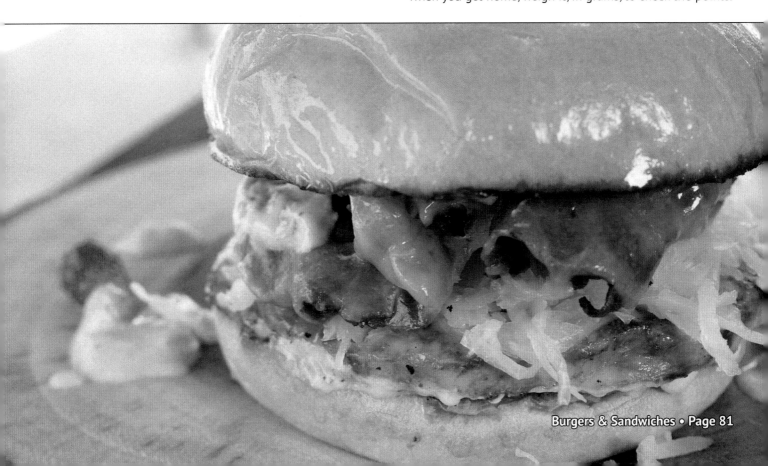

Salmon Burgers

My salmon cake appetizer, as a burger sized patty

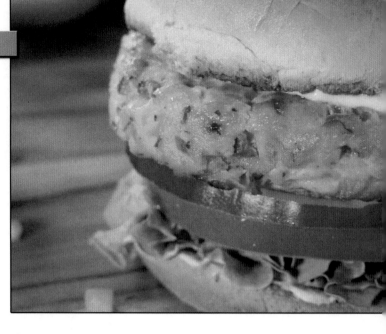

Last summer, when creating my 2nd cookbook, I heavily modified Ina Garten's famous crab cake recipe, to use salmon instead of lump crab. Ever since first making it, I always wanted to try it as a salmon burger patty, well… here we go.

Now, salmon is the highest point fish that is in the system, however, different types of salmon are different points. That information is included in the notes at the end of this recipe.

Servings Info.:
Yields: 4 sandwiches
Servings: 4
Serving Size: 1 sandwich

Points:

	G	B	P
1 serving =	5	1	1
2 servings =	10	2	2
3 servings =	14	3	3
4 servings =	19	4	4

*(These listed points **DO NOT INCLUDE** the bun. Use whichever brand buns or bread you want, then add these points. These listed points are also for using "wild pink salmon" in the WW app's database. See notes**)*

Ingredients:

- 1 pound <u>fresh or previously frozen</u> WILD, pink salmon, no skin… because that'd be gross. (see notes)
- 3 Tbsp finely diced red bell pepper
- 3 Tbsp finely diced yellow bell pepper
- 3 Tbsp finely diced red onion
- 3 Tbsp finely diced celery
- 2 Tbsp chopped flat leaf parsley
- 1/2 tsp salt
- 1/8 tsp black pepper
- 1/2 tsp old bay seasoning
- 1 egg white (2 Tbsp)
- 1/4 cup fat free Greek yogurt
- 1/2 tsp worcestershire sauce
- 1 tsp dijon mustard
- dash of hot sauce, optional
- 1 cup rice krispies style cereal. Measure the 1 cup, then crush it. You'll get over 1/2 cup crumbs for 3 points.

Lemon & White Wine Aioli:
- 3/4 cup plain fat free Greek yogurt
- 1 Tbsp light mayonnaise
- 1 Tbsp dijon mustard
- 1 Tbsp white wine (chardonnay)
- 1 tsp finely chopped dill
- 1-1/2 tsp lemon juice
- 1/4 tsp salt
- 1/8 tsp pepper
- 1/2 tsp finely chopped lemon zest (optional)

Additional Ingredients:
- Lettuce
- Tomato slices
- Sliced red onion

Directions:

1. Mix all of the Aioli ingredients together, set aside.

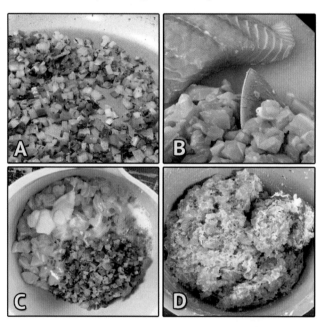

2. **(A)** Spray a pan with cooking spray, then cook the red and yellow bell peppers, red onion, celery and flat leaf parsley over medium high heat. Cook till just softened, season with salt, pepper and old bay. Set aside, allowing to cool to room temperature. **(B)** Dice all of your salmon into small bite sized chunks. You don't want perfectly uniform diced salmon, you want pieces of varying sizes. **(C)** Place the cooled vegetables, chopped salmon, egg white, yogurt, worcestershire, hot sauce and dijon mustard into a large mixing bowl. Mix until combined. **(D)** Place the rice krispies into a large ziplock bag and crush. Once they have the consistency of breadcrumbs, add all the crumbs into the salmon and mix together. Cover and allow to rest in the fridge for 30 minutes.

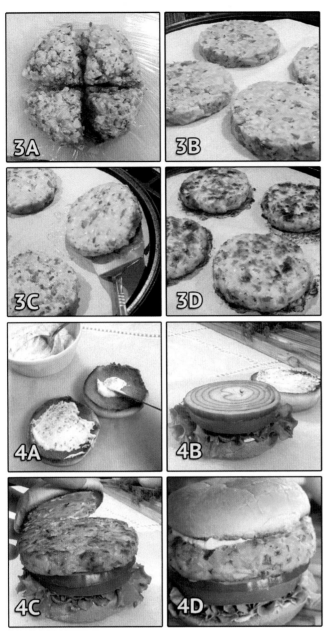

3. Preheat oven to 425 degrees.
   After the salmon has set for 30 minutes in the fridge, **(A)** divide the mix into 4 parts. **(B)** Form into 4 patties and set on a parchment paper lined baking pan. **(C)** Bake for 15 minutes at 425 degrees. Remove from oven, flip the patties, **(D)** then bake for another 15 minutes. Remove from oven.

4. To assemble the burgers, toast the buns and then **(A)** smear each with a dollop of aioli. **(B)** Place some lettuce on the spread, followed by a slice of tomato and red onion. **(C)** Place one of the salmon patties on top of the red onion and then finish with the top bun. Additionally, you can squeeze a little bit of fresh lemon juice on top of the salmon patty, prior to putting the top bun on. **(D)** Enjoy.

NOTES & SUGGESTIONS:

- *POINTS (SALMON):* This recipe uses "pink, wild, raw" salmon in the WW app. This is a little weird, because "wild atlantic salmon" is 3 points per 4oz, while "wild, pink, raw" salmon is 2 points per 4oz. So, I used wild salmon... it was pink.... so I'm saying that I used the lower point "wild, pink" salmon. Bear in mind, this ONLY matters for people on the green plan. For folks on Blue & Purple, salmon is 0 points. Greenies, use "wild, pink, raw" salmon.
- *GLUTEN:* For people rejoicing that I'm using crushed rice krispies, instead of bread crumbs... note that rice krispies brand rice cereal HAS GLUTEN. If you have a gluten sensitivity, find a brand of certified gluten free rice cereal. Use anything that will net you between 1/2 to 2/3 of crushed crumbs for 3 points.
- *DAIRY ALLERGY:* If you're allergic to dairy, you can make this recipe by substituting the yogurt for tofu in both the dressing and the patties. For the dressing, lose the mayo and blend semi firm tofu with some water until you get your desired consistency. Adjust points accordingly. The taste won't be as awesome, it'll still work. Add a little more lemon juice.

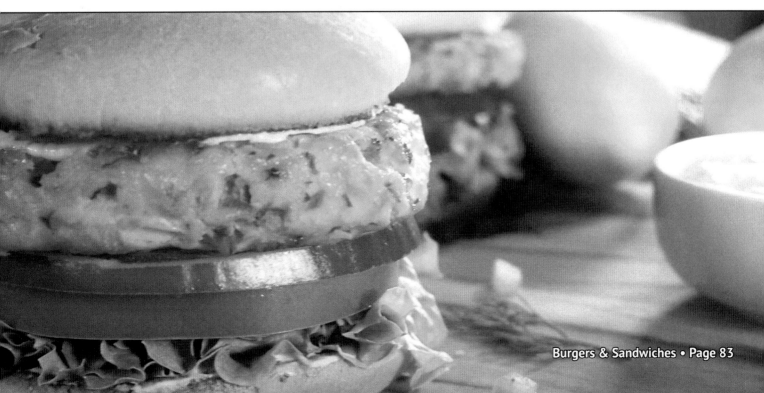

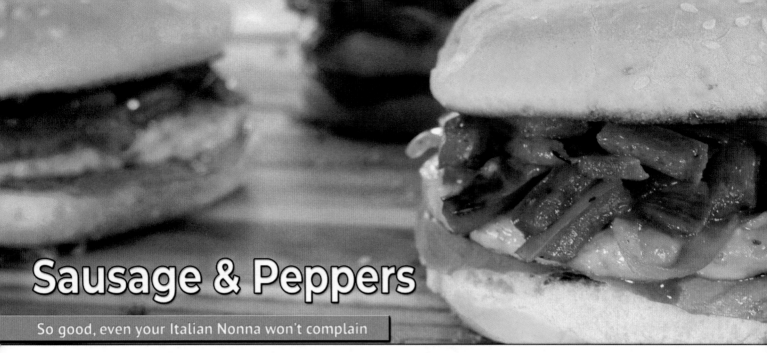

Sausage & Peppers

So good, even your Italian Nonna won't complain

One of my favorite Italian sandwiches ever is a good Italian sausage & peppers sandwich. It's typically made with links of pork Italian sausage, in casing, in a roll with cooked peppers, cheese and marinara sauce. This is my lightened up burger version, using my ground turkey Italian sausage recipe for the patties. This burger is so delicious, even **@Chiafullo** would order it, during one of his weekly sojourns to Olive Garden, for Cannoli.

Ingredients:

Savory Ground Turkey Patties
- 1/2 batch of my "Italian Sausage" ground turkey recipe, in my "Cookbook: Volume 1" on page 28, with the following changes:
    - Toast the fennel seeds, as shown in Cookbook 1, on pg. 47.

Roasted Garlic Spread
- 16-20 garlic cloves, preferably still in their skin.
- Tin foil
- Cooking spray
- 2 tsp water (trust me)

Marinara Sauce
- You can use ANY 0 point marinara sauce you want, or...
  You can make a batch of my '5 Minute Marinara', recipe on page 14.

Onions & Peppers
- 1 onion, cut into 1/4's and thin sliced
- 1 green bell pepper, cut into thin slices, then cut those in half.
- 1 red bell pepper, cut into thin slices, then cut those in half.
- salt and pepper, to taste

Additional Ingredients:
- 4 slices provolone cheese, thin sliced. You want the first slice to be 1 point, scan till you find the right brand.
- Fresh basil

Servings Info.:
Yields: 4 burgers
Servings: 4
Serving Size: 1 burger

Points:	G	B	P
1 serving =	2	1	1
2 servings =	4	2	2
3 servings =	6	3	3
4 servings =	8	4	4

*(These listed points **DO NOT INCLUDE** the bun. Use whichever brand buns or bread you want, then add these points.)*

Directions:

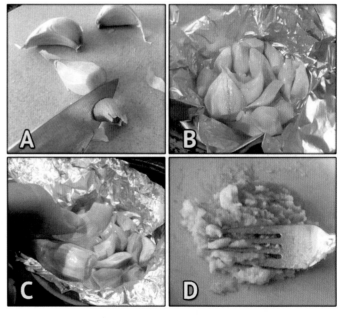

1. Preheat oven to 375 degrees. **(A)** Slice the ends off of 16-20 fresh cloves of garlic, still in the skin. **(B)** Place all of the garlic into a pouch made of tin foil, then spray with cooking spray. Close the foil pouch and bake at 375 degrees for 45 minutes. **(C)** Remove from oven, then pick up each garlic clove and gently squeeze the back end, which will cause the roasted garlic to fall out. Place all garlic cloves into a dish. **(D)** Add the water to the garlic cloves, then mash with a fork till smooth. Seal in an air tight container and set aside.

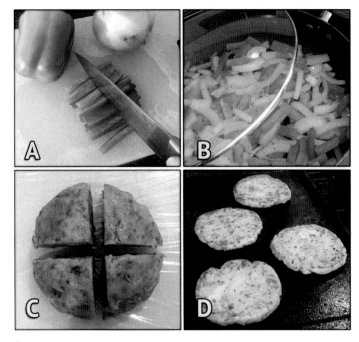

2. **(A)** Remove the seeds from the bell peppers, slice them into long thin strips, then cut those strips in half, as pictured. Quarter and then slice the onion into strips too. **(B)** Using cooking spray, cook the veggies, covered, over medium heat for 8-10 minutes. Season with salt and pepper. Turn off heat, but keep them covered. **(C)** Divide the raw meat into (4) 1/4 sections. **(D)** Form into patties and cook on both sides, then add the provolone cheese, to melt onto the patties.

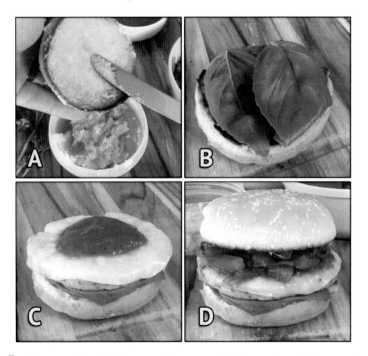

3. To assemble the burgers, first toast the buns, then **(A)** spread some of the roasted garlic onto each bun. **(B)** Place a few leaves of fresh basil onto the bottom bun, **(C)** followed by the Italian sausage patty with melted provolone. Add a dollop of marinara sauce, **(D)** then place a good amount of the cooked onions & peppers on top. Finally, cover with the top bun.

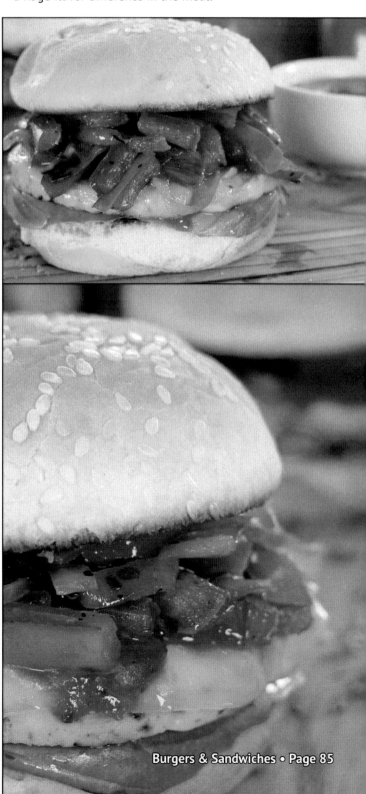

Shrimp Po'Boy

An AWESOME, healthy version of the New Orleans classic

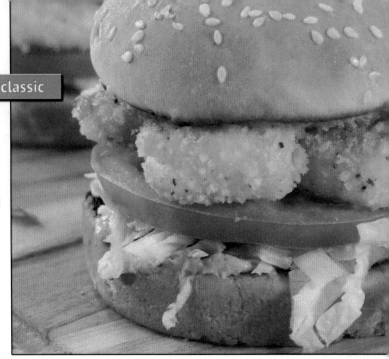

Breaded CRISPY jumbo shrimp, piled atop a thick slice of tomato, shredded lettuce... and dressed with a fan-freakin-tastic dressing. How fantastic? It's my low point, ww-ified version of the outback "blooming onion" dip, kicked up with cajun spices. It's so good it'll slap yo'momma back to the Bayou!! Though I use shrimp in this recipe, you could DEFINITELY use my breading to coat catfish, alligator, oysters, or anything you want. Make it Yo' Po'boy.

Servings Info.:

Yields: 4 sandwiches
Servings: 4
Serving Size: 1 sandwich

Points:

	G	B	P
1 serving =	2	1	1
2 servings =	5	3	3
3 servings =	7	4	4
4 servings =	9	5	5

*(These listed points **DO NOT INCLUDE** the bun. Use whichever brand buns or bread you want, then add these points. These listed points are also take the shrimp into account, for folks on the Green Plan.)*

Ingredients:

- 1 lbs X-Large (16-20 count) shrimp. Peeled, deveined, tail off. You want 20 shrimp, 5 per sandwich. **(SEE NOTES)**

Breading:

- 1 batch of my low point breading recipe, "breading 2.0", recipe in my "Cookbook: Volume 2", on pg. 35, with the following modifications:
    - Add 1 tsp cajun seasoning (in the spice aisle)
    - If you're on the Green Plan, use egg whites for the egg wash, rather than whole eggs, to reduce the points to 1 per serving, for breading.

Creole Remoulade/Dressing: (see notes)

- 2-1/2 Tbsp plain fat free Greek yogurt
- 1 Tbsp light mayonnaise
- 1 Tbsp "prepared" jarred horseradish (scan for 0 points)
- 1 Tbsp stone ground mustard (scan for a 0 point brand)
- 1 Tbsp apple cider vinegar
- 1 or 2 tsp hot sauce of choice (to taste)
- 1/4 tsp garlic powder
- 1/2 tsp smoked paprika
- 1 Tbsp no sugar added, generic ketchup (0 points)
- 1 tsp lemon juice
- 1/8 tsp salt
- 1/8 tsp black pepper
- 1/2 tsp cajun seasoning (in the spice aisle)

Additional Ingredients:

- Thin sliced/shredded Iceberg lettuce
- Tomato slices
- 20th anniversary DVD of "The Waterboy", with Bobby Bouchette.
- Optional "high quality" H20.

Directions:

1. Mix all of the Remoulade ingredients together, set aside.

2. Preheat your oven to 425 degrees. Line a large baking pan with foil and coat with cooking spray, set aside.

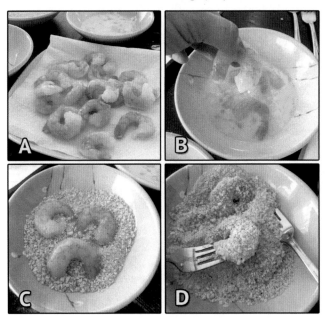

3. **(A)** Whether you buy fresh or frozen shrimp, rinse them off, then dry them with paper towels. **(B)** Dredge the shrimp in your egg wash, making sure to let the excess egg run off of each shrimp. You do NOT want tons of egg dripping into your breading and causing it to clump up. **(C)** Do NOT go the "shake and bake" route, do NOT dump all of the crumbs in a bag with the shrimp, it will not work. Place a couple of shrimp at a time into the crumbs, then **(D)** GENTLY use 2 forks, or your dry hand to lightly coat the shrimp. Repeat the process until all of your shrimp are coated. Set the shrimp onto your foil lined baking sheet.

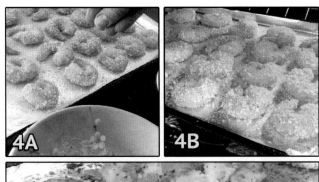

4A

4B

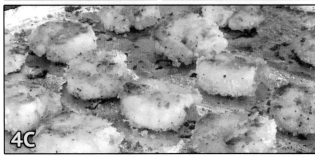

4C

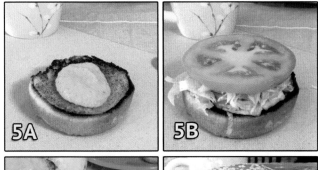

5A

5B

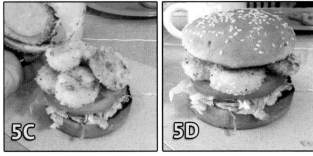

5C

5D

4. When all of the shrimp are on the pan, lightly spray them with cooking spray. **(A)** There will be a little bit of breading left, sprinkle it over all of the shrimp, to make sure they are all well coated with crumbs. Spray them with cooking spray again, then **(B)** Bake at 425 degrees for 14 minutes.
(C) Remove shrimp from oven, flip them over, then bake for an additional 2-3 minutes. Remove from oven, set aside.

5. To assemble the sandwiches, toast the buns, then **(A)** smear each one with 1 Tbsp of the Creole remoulade. **(B)** Place a mound of shredded lettuce on the spread, followed by a tomato slice. **(C)** Stack 5 pieces of shrimp on top of the tomato slice, then **(D)** place the top bun, with spread, onto the shrimp. Done.

NOTES & SUGGESTIONS:

- *SHRIMP:* You want to get shrimp that says size (16-20), 1 pound of shrimp is 4 points. This recipe calls for 5 shrimp per sandwich. Typically, bags of frozen shrimp come in 2 pound bags. I purchased a 2lb bag, pulled out 20 shrimps and called it a day.
- *DAIRY ALLERGY:* If you're allergic to dairy, you can make this recipe by substituting the yogurt and mayo for tofu in the remoulade. Replace them both with an equal amount of semi-firm tofu, blended with some water, until you get your desired consistency. Adjust points accordingly. The taste won't be as awesome, but it'll still work.
- *DRESSING:* Just a reminder, this dressing is my low calorie version of the Outback Steakhouse 'Bloomin' Onion' sauce. The only change is that I added a little bit of 'Cajun seasoning' and given it a fancy 'remoulade' name. If you want the regular Outback sauce, just remove the Cajun seasoning from the recipe.

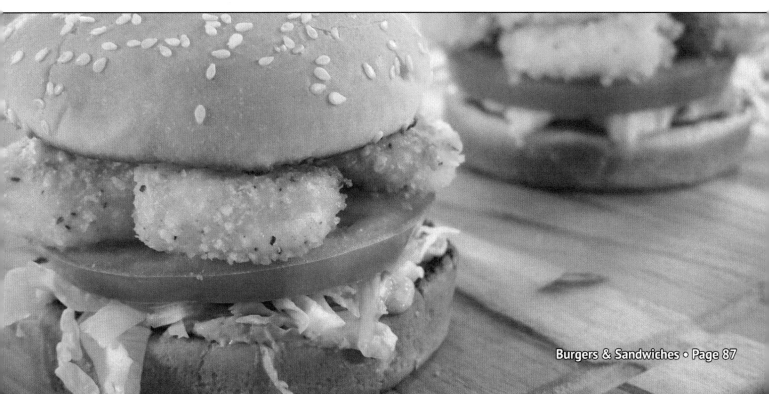

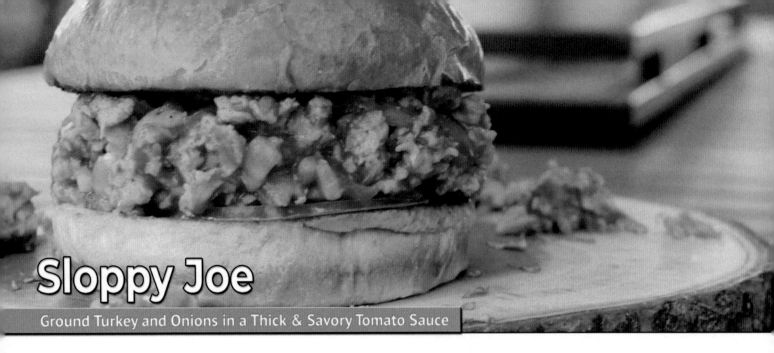

Sloppy Joe

Ground Turkey and Onions in a Thick & Savory Tomato Sauce

When I was growing up, a Sloppy Joe was pretty much some ground beef mixed with a can of 'Manwich' sauce. My lightened up recipe uses ground turkey that's heavily seasoned, with a simple tomato sauce that's tightened with a little cornstarch, instead of extra tomato paste.

Servings Info.:

Yields: 4 cups of meat.
Servings: 4
Serving Size: 1 cup

Points:

	G	B	P
1 serving =	2	0	0
2 servings =	3	0	0
3 servings =	5	0	0
4 servings =	6	1	1

(These listed points DO NOT INCLUDE the bun. Use whichever brand buns or bread you want, then add these points. This is what's between the buns)

Ingredients:

'Savory Ground Turkey':

* 1lb batch of my 'Savory' ground turkey mix, recipe in my "Cookbook: Volume 1", on page 30... with the following additions:
    - Add 2 Tbsp fat free plain Greek yogurt.
    - Add 1 Tbsp beef broth.

Sauce Ingredients:

* 1 juuuuuumbo onion, or 2 large onions, diced.
* 1 medium garlic clove, minced (fresh garlic is best)
* 15oz tomato sauce
* 1/2 cup beef broth
* 1-1/2 tsp cornstarch, dissolved with 1 Tbsp water
* additional salt and pepper, to taste.
* (optional) Thin sliced red onion. I like mine veeeery thin for this sandwich. It's purpose is to act as a barrier between the moist meat and the bottom bun. Nobody likes soggy buns. Well... at least that's what Sir Mix-a-lot says.

Directions:

1. Mix all of the ingredients together for a batch of my savory ground turkey. Then add in the diced onion and minced garlic, till well combined. Set aside for 20 minutes..

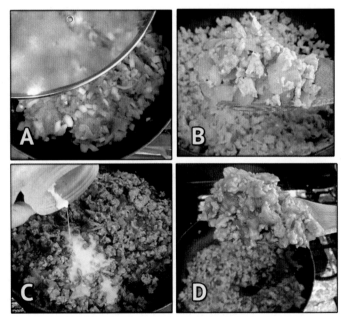

2. **(A)** Preheat a large pan for 1 minute, over medium heat. Spray the pan with cooking spray, then add the meat mixture. Cook, covered, for 10 minutes over medium heat. **(B)** Every minute or so, remove the lid and break up the meat into small pieces. When the onions are softened, remove the lid and **(C)** stir in the tomato sauce, beef broth and dissolved cornstarch. **(D)** Simmer uncovered, until most of the liquid has evaporated and the mixture has thickened. It should be around 5 minutes. Season with salt and pepper, to taste. Cover and set aside.

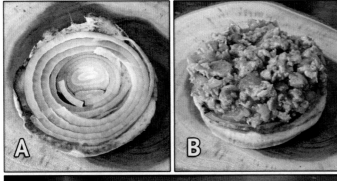

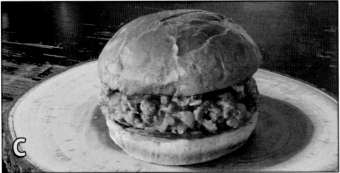

NOTES & SUGGESTIONS:

- **_NO TOMATO PASTE???:_** Every single recipe out there, for a 'sloppy joe', calls for tomato paste. It adds extra depth of flavor and thickens those 'other' sauces. Why aren't I using it? My 'Savory' ground meat mixture has so many spices and seasonings in it... that it has all the flavor we'll need. Simmering that meat mixture with the onions, garlic, beef broth and tomato sauce, gives a TON of flavor. Plus, we don't need tomato paste to tighten the sauce up. Just that tiny little bit of cornstarch will do just as well, for 0 points.

- **_RED ONION:_** Totally optional. If you're a purist that likes soggy burger buns... then leave the onions off.

- **_SLOPPY SANCHO!:_** Want to kick this baby up a notch and take it south of the border? Who needs a plain ol' Sloppy Joe?... Make a Sloppy Sancho.

  Instead of my 'Savory' meat seasoning, use my ground turkey Chorizo recipe. Buy one of those little cans of chipotle peppers in adobo sauce, then mash up one of the peppers and add it, along with a little bit of chipotle chili powder, into the tomato sauce. You can even kick it up further with some sliced jalapeños... or add some chopped, fresh cilantro under the top bun. Honestly... the Sloppy Sancho version of this sandwich is the only reason that NAFTA was ever passed.

3. **(A)** Toast your bread o' choice, then place a thin slice of red onion onto it. It won't completely stop the bun from getting soggy... but it will prolong it, as well as adding a nice textural contrast. **(B)** Add an even 1 cup scoop of the sloppy joe meat miture onto the onion. **(C)** Finally, add the top bun. Done.

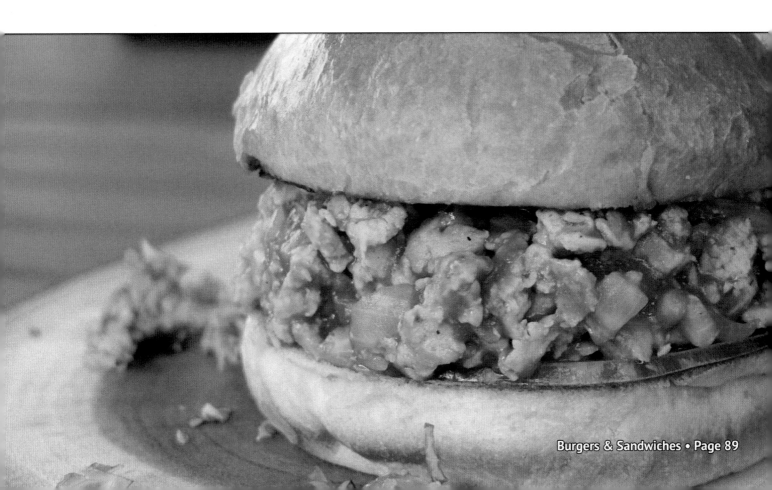

Teriyaki Pineapple

Who doesn't love pineapple and teriyaki sauce?

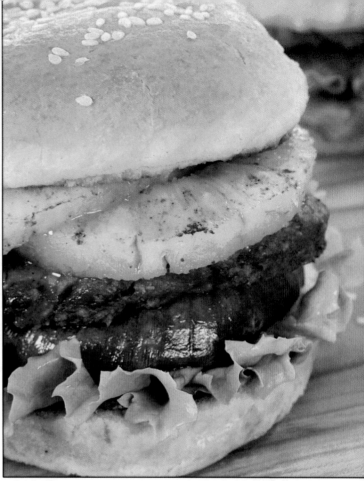

One of my favorite burgers to get at a restaurant has always been a teriyaki burger or chicken sandwich. You have a seasoned patty, savory and salty teriyaki sauce and a thick, sweet slice of pineapple. Well, we're elevating it a bit by including a roasted red onion, rather than a typical tomato, then making 2 sauces for it.

Servings Info.:	Points:	G	B	P
Yields: 4 burgers	1 serving =	1	0	0
Servings: 4	2 servings =	2	0	0
Serving Size: 1 burger	3 servings =	3	0	0
	4 servings =	4	0	0

*(These listed points **DO NOT INCLUDE** the bun. Use whichever brand buns or bread you want, then add these points.)*

Ingredients:

Savory Ground Turkey Patties
- 1/2 batch of my Savory Ground Turkey, recipe in my "Cookbook: Volume 1", on page 30.

Quick Teriyaki Sauce - *(makes 1 cup, (4) 1/4 cup servings, 0 total points.)*
- 3/4 cup water
- 2 Tbsp 0 point natural sweetener (monkfruit, stevia, etc.)**
- 1/4 tsp molasses (see notes)**
- 3 Tbsp low sodium soy sauce
- 2 Tbsp sugar free syrup (pancake syrup)
- 1 medium clove garlic, chopped
- 1/4 tsp ground ginger
- 1/8 tsp salt
- 1-1/2 tsp cornstarch, disolved in 1 Tbsp wataer
- 1/4 tsp red pepper flakes (optional)

Sesame Yogurt Dressing
- 2 Tbsp plain fat free Greek yogurt**
- 1-1/2 tsp light mayonnaise (or 2 tsp depending on brand)
- 1/4 tsp sesame oil
- 1/4 tsp ground ginger
- 1/4 tsp sriracha or other asian chili sauce (optional)
- 2 tsp of my teriyaki sauce
- 1 tsp lime juice
- pinch of salt

Additional Ingredients:
- 4 (1/2" thick) red onion slices
- 8 sliced pineapple rings, core removed.
- Chili powder and ground cinnamon, for dusting the pineapple
- Lettuce or other preferred leafy green.

Directions:

1. Mix all of the teriyaki sauce ingredients together in a small pot. Bring to a boil for 4-5 minutes, or longer if you'd like it to be thicker. Set aside.

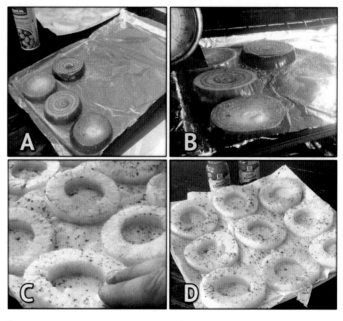

2. Preheat oven to 425 degrees. **(A)** Slice four 1/2" thick rings of red onion, then line a sheet pan with foil. Spray both sides of the onions with cooking spray and season with salt and pepper. Arrange the onions on the sheet pan, as shown. **(B)** Bake the onions at 425 for 12 minutes. **(C)** While the onions are baking, pat the pineapple rings dry with paper towels, then sprinkle with chili powder and cinnamon on 1 side. Spray rings with cooking spray, then rub the spices into the rings. **(D)** Turn the pineapple rings over, then sprinkle with more cinnamon and chili powder. Set aside.

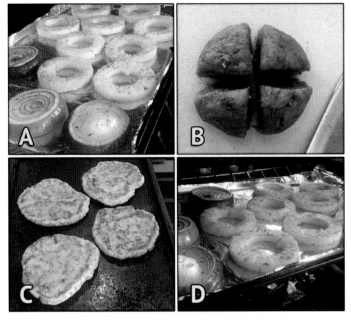

- *PINEAPPLE:* Yes, you can use canned pineapple rings instead of the fresh rings. They work, but make sure that you rinse them off, to keep them 0 points, then pat them dry with paper towels.
- Why Roasting? I never grill anything in my recipes, ever. That's because a lot of people don't have grills, so I want to accomodate them. Feel free grill the pineapple and onions, if you have access to one.
- I'm using sweetener and molasses in my teriyaki recipe, but YOU can use a 0 point brown sugar substitute instead.
- My Sesame Yogurt spread only uses 2 Tbsp of Greek yogurt, so that it stays 0 points for people on the GREEN plan. You BLUE & PURPLE folks can add another 1 Tbsp.
- If you'd like to make a full-fledge Hawaiian burger, add a slice of fried spam... but adjust your points.
- Consider making a pineapple chutney instead of the rings.

3. After 12 minutes, **(A)** remove the pan with the onions, then add the pineapple rings onto the pan. Bake for 15 more minutes. **(B)** While the pineapple and onions are baking, slice the ground turkey chorizo into 4 sections. **(C)** Form into patties and cook for 2-3 minutes per side, on medium high heat. Set aside. **(D)** Remove the baked pineapple and onions from the oven, set aside.

4. Mix together the listed ingredients for the Sesame Yogurt Dressing, set aside.

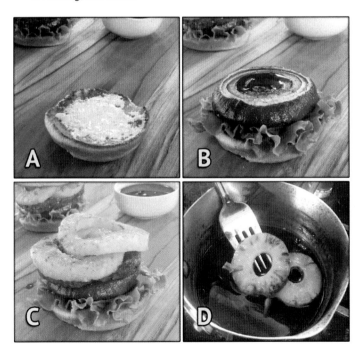

5. To assemble the burgers, first toast the buns, then **(A)** smear a scoop of the sesame dressing onto the bottom bun. **(B)** Place a layer of lettuce over the spread, followed by one of the roasted red onion rounds, covered with a bit of the teriyaki sauce. **(C)** Set a patty onto top of the onion, followed by 2 of the pineapple rings. Drizzle more teriyaki sauce over the rings, then top with the bun. **(D)** <u>OPTIONAL STEP:</u> If you want a "saucier" burger, dip your pineapple rings into the teriyaki sauce, before placing them on your burger patty.

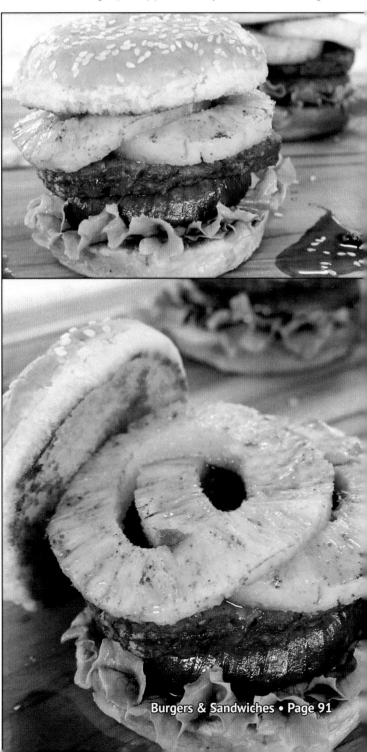

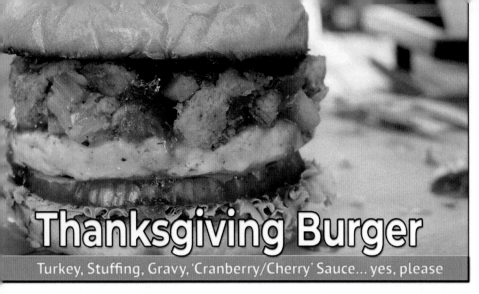

Thanksgiving Burger

Turkey, Stuffing, Gravy, 'Cranberry/Cherry' Sauce... yes, please

Servings Info.:
Yields: 4 burgers
Servings: 4
Serving Size: 1 burger

Points:	G	B	P
1 serving =	3	2	2
2 servings =	6	5	5
3 servings =	9	7	7
4 servings =	12	9	9

(These listed points DO NOT INCLUDE the bun. Use whichever brand buns or bread you want, then add these points. This is what's between the buns)

Why mope around all year, longing for Turkey Day? Now, you can have Thanksgiving on a bun year round! This burger has a patty that's loaded with fall flavors, covered in gravy and stuffing, then finished with 'cranberry' sauce.

Ingredients:

Ground Turkey Patties:
- 1/2 batch of my 'Bratwurst' recipe *(trust me)*, in my "Cookbook: Volume 1", on page 26, With the following changes:
  - Do not include the ground mustard
  - Do not include the toasted caraway seeds
  - Add 2 Tbsp plain fat free Greek yogurt

Quick Gravy:
- 3/4 cup chicken broth
- 1-1/2 tsp cornstarch
- salt and pepper to taste

Quick Dressing/Stuffing:
- 5 slices Sara Lee '45 calorie delightful' bread. *(see notes)***
- 1-1/2 cup diced onion (1 medium onion)
- 1/2 cup celery, diced
- 1/2 cup carrots, diced
- 1 medium garlic clove, chopped
- 1 tsp garlic powder
- 1-1/2 cups chicken broth
- 1 tsp onion powder
- 1/4 tsp salt
- 1/4 tsp black pepper
- 1 Tbsp fresh sage, finely chopped
- 1 Tbsp fresh rosemary, finely chopped

Faux 'Cranberry' Sauce (Dark Cherry): - see notes
- 1 cup fresh dark 'sweet' cherries, halved and pits removed.
- 1/2 cup water
- 2 Tbsp 0 point sweetener o' choice PLUS 1/4 tsp molasses, or... 2 Tbsp 0 point brown sugar substitute.
- 1/8 tsp each, ground cinnamon, ginger & nutmeg
- 2 tsp lemon juice
- 1 tsp cornstarch, dissolved with 1 Tbsp water

Additional Ingredients:
- Sliced red onion
- Preferred variety of lettuce, I used 'Green Leaf'.
- (optional) French's original fried onions *(see notes)***

1 Mix the meat and let it rest for 20 minutes. Form into 4 patties, set aside.

2 Bring the Gravy ingredients to a boil, in a small pot. Cook at a hard boil for 3 minutes. Set aside to cool.

Directions:

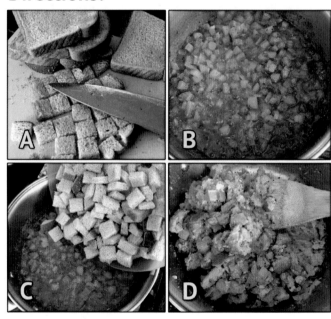

3 **(A)** Use a toaster to toast your bread, then let it sit till cool and crispy. Cut into small pieces, set aside. **(B)** In a medium sized pot, use cooking spray to sautee the onions, celery, carrots and garlic for 5-6 minutes on medium heat. Then, add the chicken broth, onion and garlic powders, salt, pepper, sage and rosemary. Simmer for 15 minutes at low heat. **(C)** Turn off the heat, and stir in the dried bread, smashing it slightly. **(D)** Cover with a lid and let sit for 10-15 minutes. Remove lid and stir, mashing it up a bit more. Season with salt and pepper to taste.

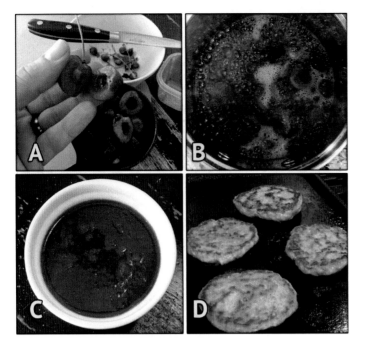

NOTES & SUGGESTIONS:
- *SLICED BREAD:* I used Sara Lee 45 calorie bread because most major stores carry it. Use whatever brand of low point bread you can find. Five slices of Sara Lee were 7 points. If you use over 7 points of bread, it will increase the points per serving by 1 point.
- *BAKED DRESSING:* If you want to bake your dressing, you can prepare it as instructed, then allow it to cool and mix in 1 whole egg. You can then bake it in the oven like traditional dressing, if you want.
- *CHERRY SAUCE???:* It was intended to be a cranberry sauce. However, cranberries are out of season and none of the stores around me even have frozen cranberries. As a result... I substituted fresh dark 'sweet' cherries in place of cranberries. When cranberries are back in season, you can use them instead. However... after trying this sauce, I will never go back to cranberry sauce, personally. This sauce is amazing. It's sweet, spiced, not very tart... it's awesome.
- *FRENCH'S FRIED ONIONS:* They are optional, but I need to mention them. If you do want to use them, sprinkle 1 Tablespoon of crunched fried onions on top of the cherry/cranberry sauce of each burger. It will add a nice crunch, while adding more Thanksgiving flair. However, if you do use them, each serving will go up 1 point.

4 **(A)** Slice the cherries in half and remove the pits. Add all of the ingredients, <u>EXCEPT FOR the cornstarch</u>, to a small pot and bring to a boil for 10 minutes. **(B)** Either blend the cherries, or mash them in the pot, till pulverized. Add the cornstarch and simmer for 3 minutes. **(C)** Set aside to cool. **(D)** Preheat a pan over medium heat for 1 minute, then spray with cooking spray. Add the patties and cook for 2 minutes per side. Set aside. Nuke the gravy in the microwave for 20 seconds or so, to quickly warm it back up.

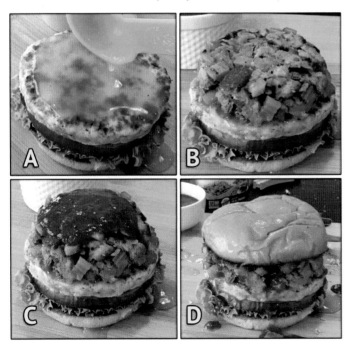

5 To assemble the sandwiches, first, toast your buns, then... **(A)** From the bottom up, place some lettuce, then a slice of red onion, followed by a turkey patty. Use a measuring spoon to scoop 2 Tablespoons of gravy onto the patty. **(B)** Measure and place 1/2 cup of dressing onto the gravy-laden patty. **(C)** Pour 2 Tablespoons of the cherry/cranberry sauce onto the stuffing, then **(D)** Cover with the top bun. Done.

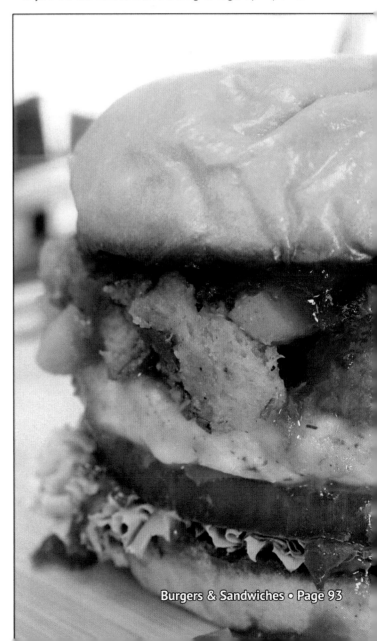

Western Bacon

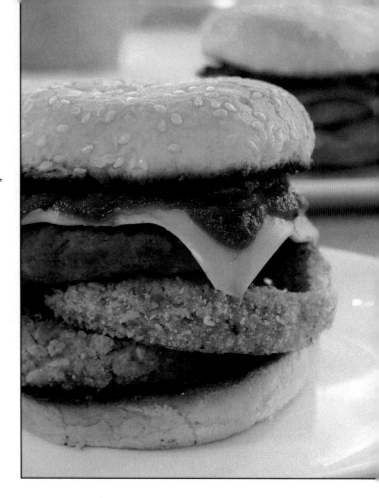

For most of my adult life, one of my favorite "chain" burgers has been the Western Bacon Cheeseburger at Carl's Jr.' but.... c'mon, the real thing is 25 points!!! So, in my never ending quest to remain a semi-skinny glutton, I had to figure out a lower calorie, lower point version of my favorite drive thru guilty pleasure.

Servings Info.:

Yields: 4 burgers
Servings: 4
Serving Size: 1 burger

Points:

	G	B	P
1 serving =	5	3	3
2 servings =	10	6	6
3 servings =	15	9	9
4 servings =	20	12	12

(These listed points DO NOT INCLUDE the bun. Use whichever brand buns or bread you want, then add these points. Points are also dependent upon your brand of cheese. These points were calculated with Borden Fat Free Cheddar singles.)

Ingredients:

Savory Ground Turkey Patties
• 1/2 batch of my Savory Ground Turkey, recipe in my "Cookbook: Volume 1", on page 30.

Quick BBQ Sauce - *(makes 2 cups, (8) 1/4 cup servings, for 1 total point)*
• Prepare a batch of my BBQ Sauce, recipe on pg. 14

Oven Baked Onion Rings
• 1 batch of my crispy oven-baked onion rings, recipe in the 'Side Dishes' section, on pg. 102

Additional Ingredients:
• 4 slices of low point american cheese slices, such as Borden's Fat Free singles (3 points), or Velveeta Original (6 points)
• 4 slices turkey bacon, uncooked, sliced in half. (see notes**)

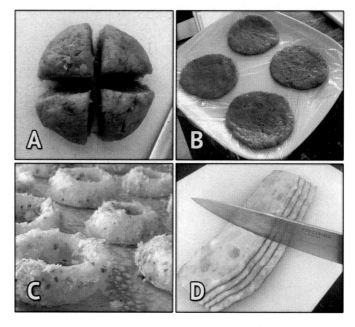

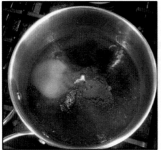 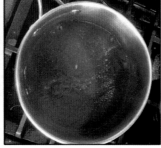

Directions:

1. Mix all of the BBQ sauce ingredients together in a small pot. Bring to a low boil, then turn off heat. Adjust seasonings as desired, set aside.

2. **(A)** Take your 1/2lb of raw "savory" ground turkey mix, then section it into 4 equal 1/4's. **(B)** Form the 4 sections into burger patties, then set aside. **(C)** Prep a batch of my onion ring appetizer recipe, then begin preheating your oven to 425 degrees. **(D)** While the oven is getting to temperature, slice the 4 strips of turkey bacon in half, then press down on the pieces with paper towels, to get them as dry as possible. It will help them get crispier when we cook them.

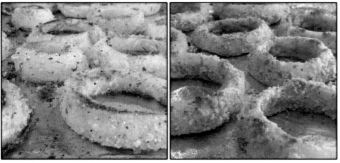

3. Once the oven comes up to temperature, spray the rings with cooking spray, then place into the oven and bake for 12 minutes at 420. After 12 minutes. Pull the onion rings out, then use a fork to flip over each ring. Return to the oven and bake for another 5-7 minutes. Set aside.

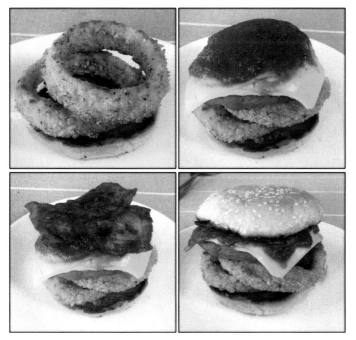

4. While the onion rings are baking, use cooking spray to cook the burger patties and halved strips of bacon. Cook the bacon to whatever your desired preference of crispness is, then melt a slice of cheese on top of the burger patties.

5. To assemble the burgers, first toast the buns. **(A)** Place 2 rings on the bottom bun, then slightly press down on them with your palm, so your patty will rest flatter on them. **(B)** Put one of the cheeseburger patties on top of the rings, topped with 1 Tbsp of BBQ sauce. **(C)** Place 2 bacon halves on top of the sauce, then **(D)** smear the top bun with a dollop of BBQ sauce and cover with the top bun. Done.

NOTES & SUGGESTIONS:

- *CHEESE:* There are 2 variables with the points for this recipe, one is the cheese. I found a Fat Free brand of cheddar cheese slices in my grocery store's cheese section, "Borden" brand, Fat Free singles. It let's you have up to 5 slices for 3 points. Velveeta Originals are the next lowest point cheese slices and they are easier to find. They will take the burgers up 1 point though.
- *BACON:* Regular turkey bacon, which is what I used, is typically 1 point per slice. If you have a Trader Joe's near you, they have a thin sliced brand of turkey bacon that lets you have 4 pieces for only 1 point.
- *BBQ Sauce:* Yes... for the love of God... I KNOW that G. Hughes makes BBQ sauce, lol. Feel free to use it if you'd like, but adjust your points accordingly.

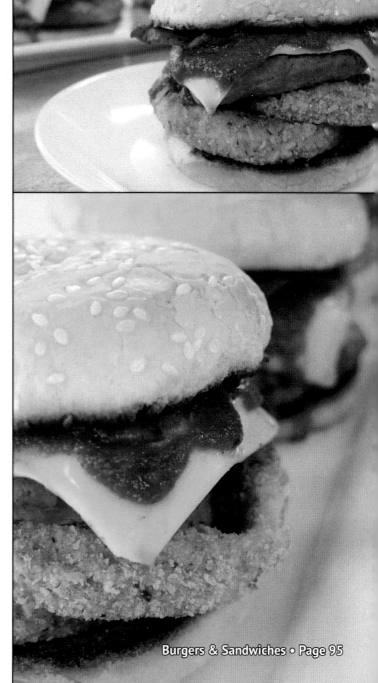

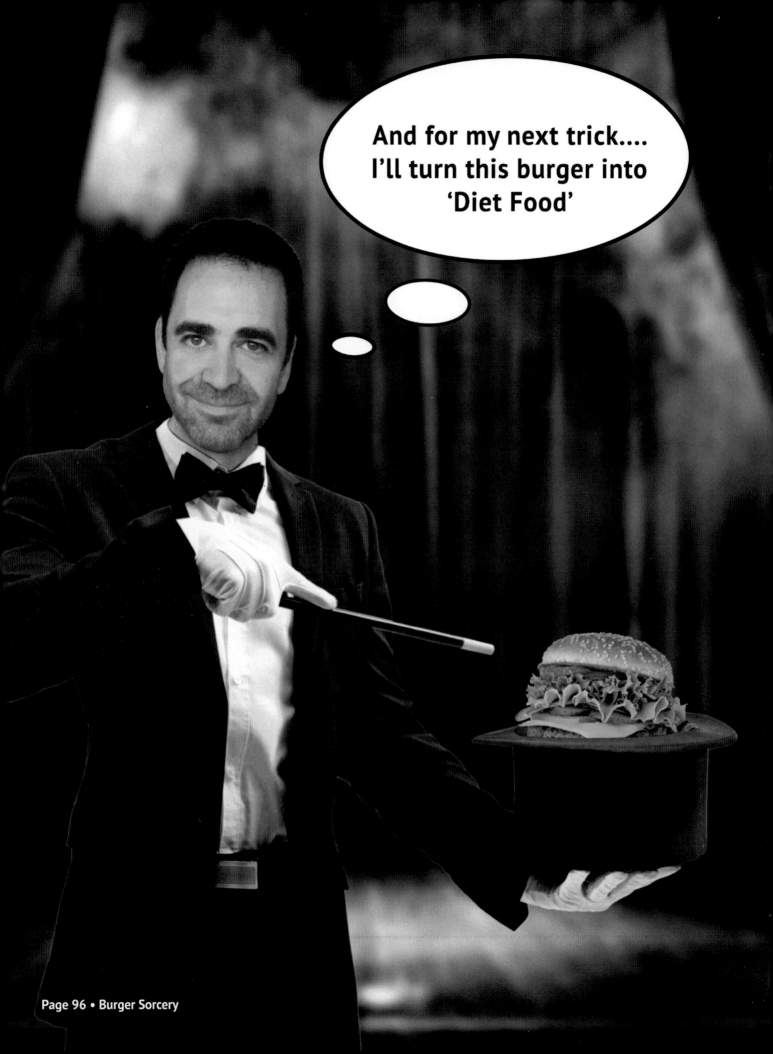

Six Points To Remember

Alright, so I just threw a head spinning amount of Gourmet, Low Calorie Burgers at you. Take a few moments and collect yourself. Take a few deep breaths, put on some Yanni, or if you live on the West Coast, like I do... proceed to one of your locally designated 'Safe Spaces'. Realize that almost everything you've been shown on major food networks, on popular food blogs... heck, even by 'celebrity chefs', for what constitutes a 'diet-friendly' burger... sucks. You DON'T have to eat sucky little plain turkey burger patties with a few veggies mixed into the meat, with 1 teaspoon of ketchup and a side of sadness. You'll notice that in the previous pages, there were no marinated tofu sliders on sandwich thins. My goal is to let you eat big, satisfying, macho portions of food that'll convert even the stubborn people in your family that refuse to eat your 'diet food'. We'll convert'em.

#1. Again, I want to reiterate that you do NOT have to use 99% fat free ground turkey like I did. I only used it because of it's 'Points' value within Weight Watchers. The awesome thing is, because I have developed all of my burgers to be so absolutely low in calories and fat, if you want to use 93% ground turkey, or if you want to use extra lean ground beef... YOU CAN. Use what you'd like. Use those meats and your burgers will STILL be extremely low in calories, fat and 'Points'. My recipes are a guide/template for you to customize to your liking.

#2. If you DO use beef with my seasoning mixes... do NOT add the chicken or beef bouillon/granules. They are used to add more savory flavor to ground turkey and chicken. Ground beef doesn't need it. Same goes with ground cumin. If you are using ground beef with my seasoning mixes, ONLY include the cumin with the Chorizo and Cuban Picadillo recipes. Ground cumin helps mask the distinctive turkey flavor. In the Chorizo and Picadillo, it's essential for the 'Latin' flavor.

#3. *MOIST BURGERS:* Remember, if you are using extremely lean ground meat and you want to add a little more moisture to it... mix in 1 Tbsp of plain fat free Greek yogurt. Why is 99% fat free ground turkey and 98% fat free ground beef so dry? They're missing fat. What is Fat? It's thick, white and creamy. What is plain fat free Greek yogurt? Thick, white and creamy. *lightbulb*

#4. Remember... for your patties. If you are using 99% fat free ground turkey or ground chicken... whether you are cooking them on a hot pan or a hot grill... they cook extremely fast because of the lack of fat. If you are cooking thin patties, preheat the pan over medium-high heat for 1 minute, then cook the patties for 2 minutes per side. If you are cooking 1/4 pound patties, 3 minutes per side. Because of the baking soda trick (TRUST ME ON USING IT), if you cook your meat too long, it gets a very thin firm outer layer of meat to it.

#5. Remember, my recipes are for what goes 'between' the buns/bread. All of the nutritional info for every recipe is in the back of this book. Add the calories, fat and 'Points' of my recipe to whateeeeeever bread or bun you use for your burger. My burgers are so low in those 3 things that you can even use a big ol' bakery pretzel bun, and it'd still be pretty danged healthy.

#6. Most important... Just because these are low calorie, low fat and low 'Point' burgers, does not mean you should gorge on them. Eat mindfully. If you go to Red Robin, you are NOT going to order 2 gigantic burgers and expect to not gain weight. This is the same thing. I have developed these to be big, satisfying burgers... that just happen to be low in calories (compared to regular, similar burgers). Eat one of these big monsters... and move on with your day. Eat mindfully, use your head, and by the end of the day you will have eaten delicious, filling food, and still end the day in a calorie deficit, while not starving yourself.

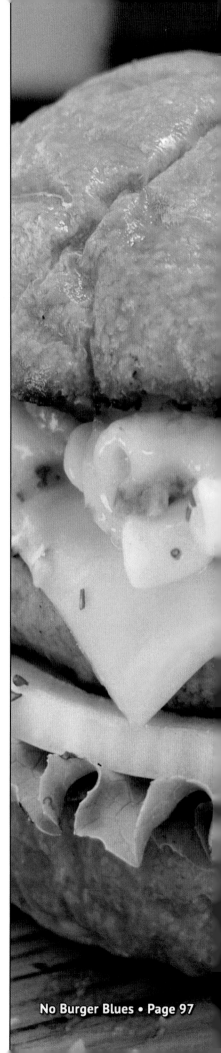

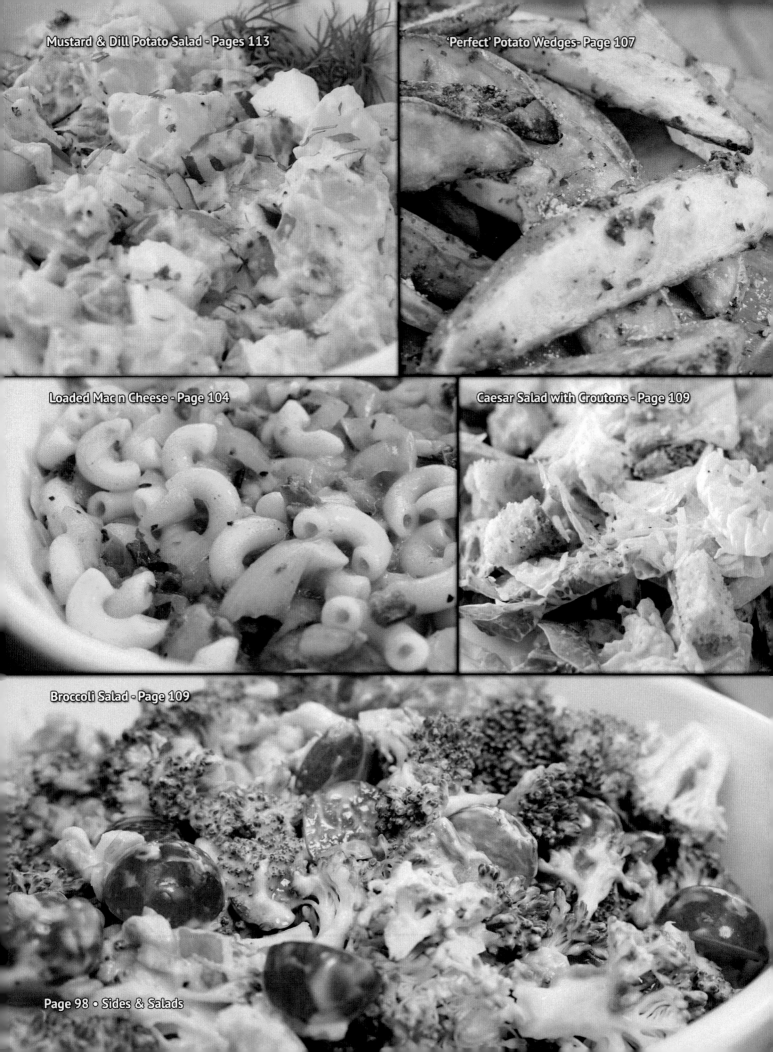

Mustard & Dill Potato Salad - Pages 113

'Perfect' Potato Wedges- Page 107

Loaded Mac n Cheese - Page 104

Caesar Salad with Croutons - Page 109

Broccoli Salad - Page 109

Sides & Salads

A small collection of low fat, low calorie, low 'Point' side dishes and salads that would pair well with my burgers and sandwiches.

Sides

Balsamic Glazed Brussel Sprouts ····· Pg. 100
Creamed Style Sweet Corn ··········· Pg. 101
Crispy Baked Onion Rings ··········· Pg. 102
Garlic Dijon Mushrooms ··········· Pg. 103
Loaded Mac n Cheese ··········· Pg. 104
Maple & Bacon Baked Beans ········ Pg. 105
Parmesan Carrot Fries ··········· Pg. 106
Perfect Potato Wedges ··········· Pg. 107

Salads

BBQ Ranch Chicken Salad ··················· Pg. 108
Blue Cheese Wedge Salad ·················· Pg. 108
Broccoli Salad ························· Pg. 109
Caesar Salad ························· Pg. 109
Classic Creamy Coleslaw ················· Pg. 110
Cobb Salad ······················· Pg. 110
Creamy Roasted Garlic & Onion Pasta Salad ··· Pg. 111
Crunchy Asian Chicken Salad ··············· Pg. 111
Mediterranean Salad (Olive Garden) ·············· Pg. 112
Mexican 'Street Corn' Salad ············· Pg. 112
Mustard & Dill Potato Salad ··········· Pg. 113

Bonus Recipes

Burger Buns (yeast) ················ Pg. 114-115
Cucumber Mint Lemonade ·········· Pg. 116
Easy Peach Cobbler ················ Pg. 117
Peanut Butter & Jelly Cake ········· Pg. 118-119
Personal Sized Cocoa Cake ········· Pg. 120-121
    - Plus 7 flavor variations

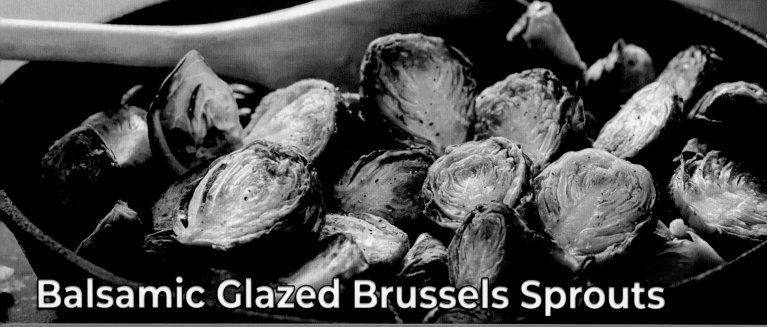

Balsamic Glazed Brussels Sprouts

Pan seared Brussels sprouts with a balsamic glaze, finished with reduced fat parmesan topping

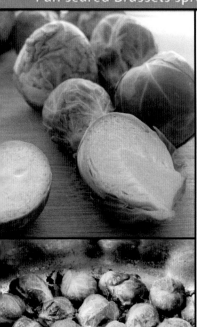

I need to start off by admitting that I never ate Brussels sprouts, even once, until I was married. I decided to try cooking them at home for my wife, shortly after we got hitched. Let's just say that I overcooked them so bad that it was 14 years before I EVER tried cooking them again. This recipe has redeemed my faith in these little cabbage-like balls. It comes together quickly, with a finished dish that is savory, sweet, has a slight vinegary pop and a mildly earthy flavor. Plus... it's pretty.

Ingredients:

- 1-1/2 pounds Brussels sprouts
- Flavored cooking spray o' choice. I used butter flavored, scan to ensure a 0 point amount is used.
- 1/4 tsp salt
- 1/8 tsp pepper
- 2 Tbsp balsamic vinegar
- 1 Tbsp red wine vinegar
- 1 Tbsp reduced fat parmesan topping, like the old-school 'Kraft' brand sprinkles. *(optional)*

Serving Info.:

Yields: 6 cups
Servings: 4
Serving Size: 1.5 cup

Points:

	G	B	P
1 serving =	1	1	1
2 servings =	2	2	2
3 servings =	2	2	2
4 servings =	3	3	3

Directions:

1 Carefully cut off the very end of each Brussels sprout, leaving most of it intact. Leaving a bit of the end intact will help the lil mini cabbage-like grenades, stay together while they cook.
2 Next, carefully slice each one in half, as pictured to the left (top picture).
3 Heat a large pan over medium heat for 1 minute, so that it gets nice and hot. You want water droplets to evaporate instantly upon hitting it. Spray the pan with a 0 point amount of your cooking spray. Place Brussels sprouts, flat side down, onto the hot pan, crank up the heat to medium-high and cook for about 3-5 minutes, till they brown. Just let them sit there and sear, don't stir them all around the pan. Be sure to not overcrowd them, or they'll steam, which can make them bitter and taste like a camel's backside... don't ask. If all the sprouts don't fit in the pan at once, sauté them in two batches.
4 Season with some of the salt and pepper, then, rotate them onto their other side. Season with the remaining salt and pepper, then cook for 2-3 more minutes.
5 Combine the two vinegars, then pour them into the pan. Gently stir the sprouts around, to coat in the liquid. Cook for 1-2 more minutes, until the vinegar reduces and glazes the sprouts.
6 Sprinkle parmesan topping over all the sprouts, toss to coat. Done.

Note:

- Feel free to use regular parmesan cheese, but adjust your points accordingly.
- The Brussels sprouts should NOT be mushy. If they overcook, they get very bitter... and then you won't eat them again for 14 years. Trust me, don't over cook Brussels sprouts.
- Forgot to mention... I've only made these with fresh Brussels sprouts, I haven't tried it with frozen ones. You'd most likely need to thaw them out first and try to pat them dry with paper towels. Cook time would probably need to be increased as well.
- You can also amp these up by adding cooked and crumbled turkey bacon. But, adjust the points if you do.

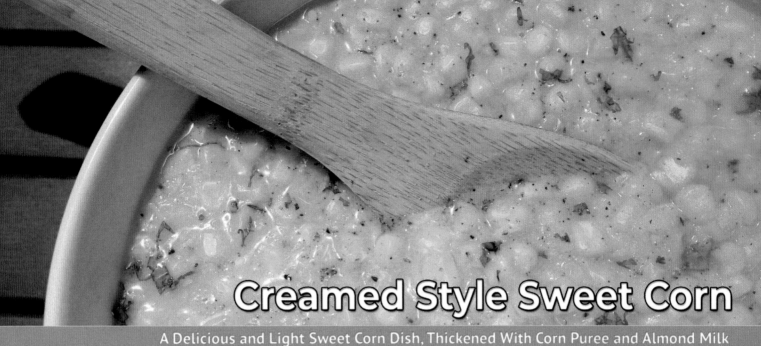

Creamed Style Sweet Corn

A Delicious and Light Sweet Corn Dish, Thickened With Corn Puree and Almond Milk

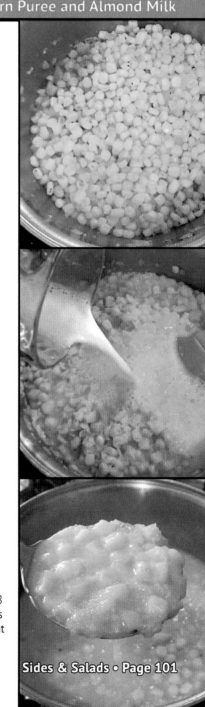

Growing up, I used to eat canned creamed corn whenever I could, I loved it. Not until I grew up and had to join weight watchers, did I start paying attention to how much fat, calories and sugar were in a typical can. My version uses a couple of tricks to thicken up and get creamy. One: Like my cornbread muffin recipe, I blend 1 can of corn, then add that in as a thickener. Two: Instead of half n half or whole milk, I use unsweetened almond milk, with a little dissolved cornstarch, which will thicken up as it simmers.

Ingredients:

- Butter flavored cooking spray
- 1/2 cup diced onions
- 1/2 tsp salt
- 1/4 tsp pepper
- (2) 15oz cans whole kernel corn, drained.
- *** (18oz by weight, for the 2 cans worth of corn, drained)
- 2 Tbsp 0 point sweetener o' choice
- (1) 15oz can whole kernel corn, blended with it's liquid.
- 1 cup unsweetened plain almond milk**
- 1-1/2 tsp cornstarch, dissolved into water

Serving Info.:

Yields: 4-1/2 cups
Servings: 9
Serving Size: 1/2 cup

Points:

	G	B	P
1 serving =	3	0	0
2 servings =	6	0	0
3 servings =	9	0	0
4 servings =	12	0	0

Directions:

1 Heat a medium sized pot over medium heat for 1 minute. Spray with a good amount of butter flavored cooking spray (make sure it's a 0 point amount), then add the onions, salt and pepper. Cook over medium heat for 3 minutes.
2 Add the 2 cans of drained corn, along with the sweetener. Cook for 5 minutes.
3 Add the blended can of corn. Mix the almond milk, water and cornstarch, then pour into the pot.
4 Bring it all up to a light boil, then reduce heat to medium-low. Simmer for 30 minutes. Done.

Note:

- GREENIES: Rather than adding the points for 30oz of corn, from the 2 whole kernel cans, I drained the corn, THEN weighed it. Drained, the 2 cans gave 18.5oz of corn, which is what I input into the recipe. 30oz of corn is 24 points, 18.5oz is 15. To those 15 points, I added 12 points for the can of blended corn. It saved the points from 11.5 oz. Sorry for the techo-mumbo-jumbo... it's a Green-thing.
- Most creamed corn recipes call for a TON of half n half or whole milk. We're completely eliminating those. In order to get the creamy consistency, we're mixing in blended corn and the almond milk, which will thicken with the cornstarch.
- When you 'blend' the 1 can of corn, do not completely puree it to liquid. You want to leave it slightly pulpy and thick.
- If you are allergic to almond milk, you can use soy milk or skim milk, but adjust your points.
- Some brands of butter flavored cooking spray let you use more before they get points. Some let you have 8 seconds of spray for 0 points, other let you paint a Buick with it for 0. The brand that I use (vons/albertsons ralphs/kroger Signature brand) stays 0 points, period... I use a good 6 second burst. Scan your can, use what you can. It really does add a nice buttery flavor, for no additional fat or calories.

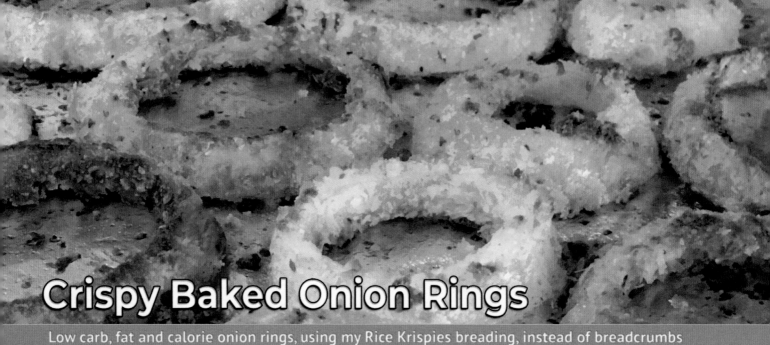

Crispy Baked Onion Rings

Low carb, fat and calorie onion rings, using my Rice Krispies breading, instead of breadcrumbs

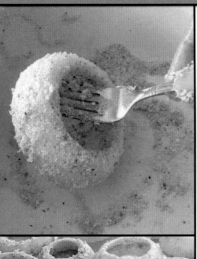

Though not speciiiiifically mentioned in the Good Book... real, crispy, gloriously low point, onion rings are something worthy of a choir of Angels. Instead of breadcrumbs, we're crushing up Rice Krispies cereal... just go with it. It's lower in calories, carbs, points and keeps a nearly identical texture to regular breadcrumbs. People with Gluten allergies can use gluten free rice cereal.

Ingredients:

- 2 large onions, sliced into 1/2" thick rings

Breading:
- 1-1/4 cup crispy rice cereal (like rice krispies). Place it in a ziplock bag and crush it. You'll end up with right around 2/3 cup.
- 1-1/2 tsp plain breadcrumbs
- 2 tsp panko breadcrumbs
- 1/4 tsp salt
- 1/4 tsp black pepper
- 1/4 tsp garlic powder
- 1/4 tsp onion powder
- 1/2 tsp italian seasoning

Egg Wash:
- 2 large eggs (or egg whites, for Greenies)
- 1-1/2 tsp self rising flour
- 1-1/2 tsp cornstarch
- 1 tsp dijon mustard
- 1 Tbsp water

Serving Info.:

Yields: 6 cups
Servings: 4
Serving Size: 1.5 cup

Points:

	G	B	P
1 serving =	1	1	1
2 servings =	2	2	2
3 servings =	3	3	3
4 servings =	4	4	4

Directions:

1 Mix the breading ingredients and set in a large bowl. For the egg wash, first mix the flour, cornstarch, mustard and water, till smooth. Whisk together the eggs in a bowl, then add the dijon mixture. Set aside.
2 Preheat oven to 425 degrees. Line a baking sheet pan with foil, spray with cooking spray, set aside.
3 Slice the onions, then ONE AT A TIME, dip each ring into the egg wash. Use 1 hand to lift the ring out of the egg wash, and allow extra egg to fall back into the bowl. Place the egg-coated ring into the bowl with the rice cereal crumbs. Use a fork to lightly toss crumbs onto the ring, lightly coating it. Place onto the prepared baking sheet. Repeat for EVERY INDIVIDUAL RING. Do not try breading them all together!
4 Coat the onion rings with cooking spray, bake at 425 degrees for 15 minutes. Remove from oven, flip the rings, spray with cooking spray, bake for 10 more minutes, or until golden. Done.

NOTES:
- Listed points for the Green plan assume you are using egg whites, rather than whole eggs.

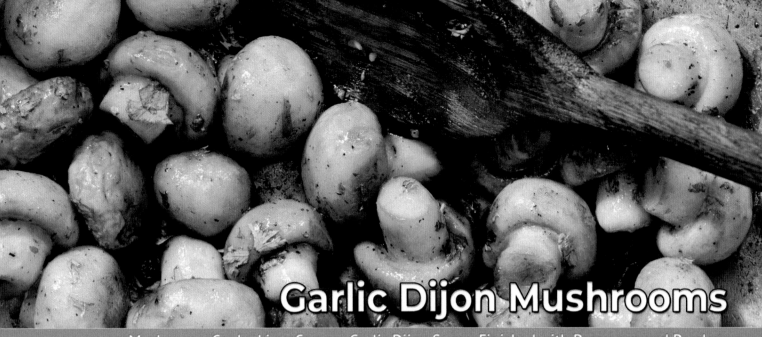

Garlic Dijon Mushrooms

Mushrooms Cooked in a Creamy Garlic Dijon Sauce, Finished with Parmesan and Parsley

So, in this recipe, we're going to commit culinary blasphemy by replacing the butter that NORMAL recipes call for, with a good spray of butter flavored cooking spray. Ya'll know me well enough after two cookbooks to know that's my thing. We're then coating them in a sauce of reduced chicken broth, garlic and a little dijon mustard. Finally, to add an extra punch of savory flavor, we're adding reduced fat Parmesan.

Ingredients:

- (3) 8oz packages whole mushrooms, any preferred variety. Washed, dried, ends trimmed.
- Butter flavored cooking spray (see notes)***
- 4 medium cloves garlic, crushed, chopped
- 1/4 tsp salt
- 1/4 tsp pepper
- 1/3 cup beef broth
- 2 tsp dijon mustard
- 1/2 tsp cornstarch dissolved with 1 Tbsp water
- 1 Tbsp reduced fat parmesan topping (like the Kraft brand)
- 2 Tbsp finely chopped parsley or rosemary

Serving Info.:

Yields: 3 cups
Servings: 4
Serving Size: 3/4 cup

Points:

	G	B	P
1 serving =	0	0	0
2 servings =	1	1	1
3 servings =	1	1	1
4 servings =	1	1	1

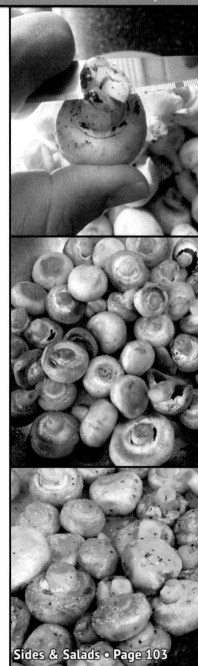

Directions:

1. Wash and lightly scrub the mushrooms, removing as much dirt as possible. Rinse the mushrooms, **DON'T** submerge them and walk away, think of them as little sponges. Slice off the end of the stalks, set the mushrooms aside.
2. Heat a large pan over medium-high heat for 1 minute. Spray with a goooood amount of 0 point butter flavored cooking spray, then add the mushrooms, salt and pepper. Cook for 3 minutes.
3. Once browned and lightly seared, stir in 1/3 cup beef broth and garlic. Continue cooking, over medium-high heat, for another 3 minutes.
4. Mix the dijon mustard into the dissolved cornstarch. Add to the pan and stir to combine. Cook for an additional 2-3 minutes, or until the mushrooms have darkened, have cooked down a bit and are covered in a nice thick coating of sauce. Turn off the heat and sprinkle with 1/2 the Parmesan, stir to combine. Taste and season with additional salt and pepper, if needed.
5. Plate the mushrooms in a large communal bowl, or serve in (4) 8 ounce ramekins. Garnish with fresh parsley and the remaining Parmesan.

Note:

- I purchased packages of whole white button mushrooms from my local grocery store. However, if you want to get all 'fancy Nancy', go ahead and buy Crimini mushrooms.
- If you've never cleaned mushrooms before and the sound of it's a little intimidating, watch a youtube video. That's what I did. It's really simple.
- Butter Flavored Cooking Spray?!?!: Yup, trust me. Scan your can to see how much you can use to stay at 0 points. I was able to use a solid 8 second buttery spray. It gave a great butter flavor to the dish. Cry me a river, foodie-hipsters! I'm cutting calories.
- If you're having a heart attack at the thought of using Kraft Parmesan sprinkles... go ahead and use real Parmesan, but adjust your points, Nancy.
- If you aren't a fan of mustard, feel free to replace it with a little bit of extra broth, or 2 tsp balsamic vinegar.

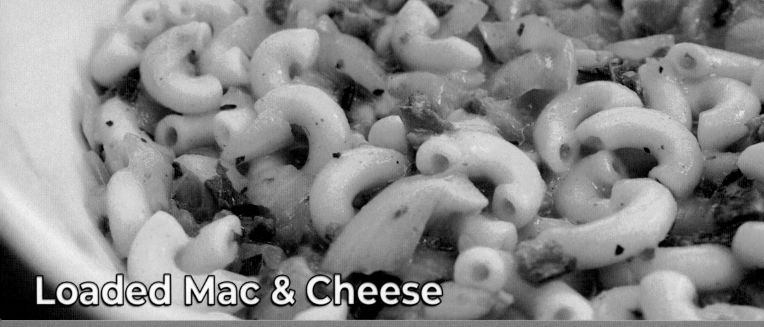

Loaded Mac & Cheese

Mac n cheese with my low fat cheese sauce, turkey bacon crumbles, caramelized onions and kale

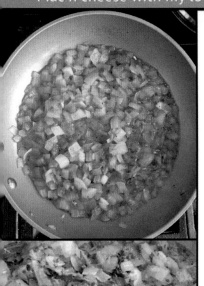

This is my version of a low calorie and low fat mac n cheese, that DOES NOT REQUIRE CAULIFLOWER!!!! Praise Jesus! We're using my quick cheese sauce, from the mac n cheese burgers, then pairing it with some caramelized onions, garlic, crispy chopped turkey bacon and some chopped kale for a little crunch and color. I decided to add a little smoked paprika to give it that little smoky flavor, as well as depth.,

Ingredients:

- 1-1/3 cup elbow macaroni pasta, cooked, set aside.
- 2 strips turkey bacon, cooked with spray, set aside.
- 1 large onion, diced
- 1 medium clove garlic, chopped
- 3/4 cup beef broth
- 1/4 tsp each, salt, pepper, onion powder and smoked paprika
- 1/2 cup finely chopped kale or preferred green leafy veggie, such as spinach, swiss chard, etc.
- 1 batch of my cheese sauce, recipe on pg. 15.
- dash of hot sauce, optional

Serving Info.:

Yields: 2-1/2 cups
Servings: 5
Serving Size: 1/2 cup

Points:

	G	B	P
1 serving =	3	3	1*
2 servings =	5	5	2*
3 servings =	8	8	4*
4 servings =	10	10	5*

Directions:

1. Precook the macaroni pasta and crispy bacon. Set them aside for later.
2. Heat pan over medium heat for 1 minute, then add the diced onions and garlic. Add in beef broth, salt, pepper, onion powder, smoked paprika and hot sauce (if using). Cover with a lid, bring to a low boil and allow to cook for 14-15 minutes, till most of the liquid evaporates. Turn off heat.
3. Stir in the chopped bacon and kale, stir to combine, replace lid, set aside so that it can steam the kale for a few minutes.
4. Prepare the cheese sauce, as directed in the recipe.
5. In medium pot, combine the cooked pasta, bacon & onion mixture and the cheese sauce.
6. Turn on the heat, bring to a simmer and allow to bubble for 1-2 minutes. Done.

Note:

- The points listed are calculated with Fat Free cheese slices in the sauce. If you use higher point/calorie/fat cheese slices, adjust your points accordingly.
- Use whatever brand of bacon you wish. The brand of turkey bacon that I used was 2 points for 2 slices. Some brands allow you to have more bacon for 2 points. If you'd like to use regular pork bacon, use center cut.
- Points for the **PURPLE** plan, are shown as if you are using whole wheat, or not 'enriched flour' elbow macaroni... or any 0 point type of elbow macaroni.

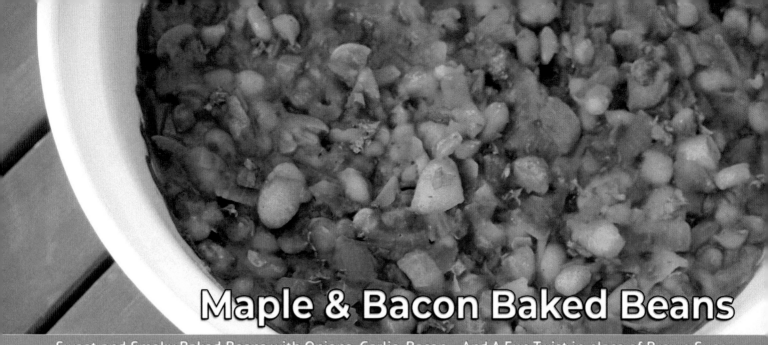

Maple & Bacon Baked Beans

Sweet and Smoky Baked Beans with Onions, Garlic, Bacon... And A Fun Twist in place of Brown Sugar

Whenever I go to a BBQ place and get a sandwich, I ALWAYS order baked beans as a side. I've made them a few times over the years, but most recipes always require a ton of brown sugar or molasses. I used to use an equally large amount of artificial brown sugar substitute instead. However, I recently came across a recipe that uses root beer in place of all of it. I decided to go about WW-erizing it, to make it lower in calories, while adding some other twists to it. It turned out really well. It has a subtle smoky flavor, with a slight hint of caramel.

Ingredients:

- 2 slices turkey bacon
- 1 large onion, diced
- 1 medium garlic clove, minced
- 1/4 cup tomato sauce
- 12oz diet root beer***
- 1 Tbsp apple cider vinegar
- 1 Tbsp sugar free maple syrup (pancake syrup)
- 1/4 tsp ground mustard
- 1/2 tsp smoked paprika
- 1/4 tsp molasses (optional)
- (2) 15oz cans (or a 30oz can), cannellini beans, drained and well rinsed. Once drained, it's 16oz of actual beans.
- 1/2 tsp salt
- 1/4 tsp pepper

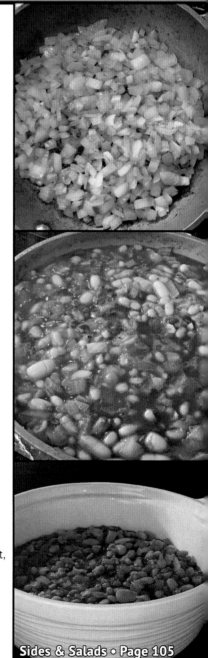

Serving Info.:

Yields: 3 cups
Servings: 4
Serving Size: 3/4 cup

Points:

	G	B	P
1 serving =	3	1	1
2 servings =	5	1	1
3 servings =	8	2	2
4 servings =	10	2	2

Directions:

1 Preheat oven to 400 degrees. While it's heating: In a large pan, use cooking spray to cook the bacon until crispy, remove from pan. Spray pan with cooking spray again, then add the onion and cook till they begin to soften. 3-4 minutes.
2 Stir in the garlic and cook for 1-2 minutes, till fragrant. Add the tomato sauce, root beer, vinegar, syrup, ground mustard, smoked paprika, molasses (if using), salt and pepper. Stir to combine, return to a boil.
3 Gently stir in the beans and crumbled bacon. Bring it to a simmer, then reduce the heat to medium-low and cook, uncovered for 18 minutes, stirring occasionally.
4 Pour the beans into a 1-1/2 quart, oven-safe casserole dish. Bake uncovered at 400 degrees for 30 minutes, or until the beans & sauce have thickened. Season with additional salt and pepper to taste.

Note:

- GREENIES... weigh your beans! If you simply look up 30oz of canned cannellini beans, it's 16 points. But if you actually open that 30oz can of beans, drain, rinse, then weigh them, it's really 16 oz of beans, by weight, which is only 8 points.
- I use sugar free pancake 'maple' syrup because I don't have food sensitivities to it. Plus, 1 Tbsp of any brand is 0 points. Feel free to use regular maple syrup if you wish, but adjust your points.
- The brand of turkey bacon I used is 1 point per slice, for a total of 2 points. Use whatever brand or type of bacon you prefer. Some brands let you have a lot more bacon for 2 points than others do.

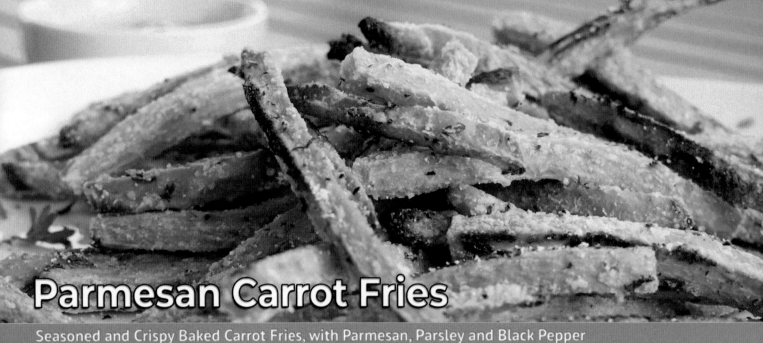

Parmesan Carrot Fries

Seasoned and Crispy Baked Carrot Fries, with Parmesan, Parsley and Black Pepper

These tasty little carrot sticks would make Bugs Bunny hug Elmer Fudd, out of joy. We're switching up the idea of baked regular fries and using a healthier and lower calorie alternative... carrots. To save time, we're buying pre cut carrot sticks from the produce department. Then, we're seasoning them with some salt, pepper, garlic powder, reduced fat parmesan and parsley. Cooking spray replaces a bunch of oil, then 'Voila'... healthy fries.

Ingredients:

- 1.5lbs (2 12oz bags) packaged carrot sticks. Or... feel free to cut your own from fresh carrots. You do you, boo.
- 0 point coating of cooking spray. Use whatever flavor spray you want, scan your can, use a 0 point amount.
- 1/4 tsp olive oil
- 1 tsp garlic powder
- 1 tsp onion powder
- 1/2 tsp salt
- 1/4 tsp pepper
- 1-1/2 tsp cornstarch
- 1 Tbsp reduced fat parmesan topping (such as 'Kraft' brand)
- 1 Tbsp fresh parsley, finely chopped, packed

Serving Info.:

Yields: 1 pound
Servings: 4
Serving Size: 1/4 pound

Points:

	G	B	P
1 serving =	0	0	0
2 servings =	1	1	1
3 servings =	1	1	1
4 servings =	1	1	1

Directions:

1 Preheat oven to 425 degrees. Line 2 large cookie sheet pans with parchment paper, set aside.
2 Place carrot sticks into a large mixing bowl. Add the 1/4 tsp olive oil and spray the carrots liberally with cooking spray. Make sure to use only enough cooking spray to stay 0 points.
3 In a small bowl, mix together the garlic powder, onion powder, salt, pepper, cornstarch, parmesan and parsley. Pour the seasoning mixture into the bowl with the carrots, toss till well combined.
4 Spread the carrots onto the parchment paper lined baking pans, in a single layer.
5 Bake at 425 degrees for 35 minutes, depending on desired texture. Remove from oven.
6 Garnish with additional fresh chopped parsley, if desired.

Note:

- If you'd like them to have a little sweetness, feel free to add a little bit of sweetener into the mix of seasonings.
- This recipe is highly customizable. Want things a little Latin? Add some chili powder or cumin. For an exotic flavor, try adding a little curry powder and maybe a dash of ground ginger. Have fun with it.
- Feel free to try decreasing the cooking time, by increasing the temperature to 450 degrees. They'll cook faster, but you'll have to keep an eye on them, to make sure they don't burn.

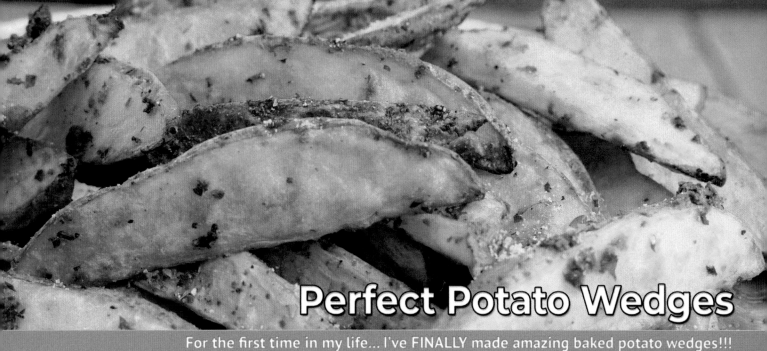

Perfect Potato Wedges

For the first time in my life... I've FINALLY made amazing baked potato wedges!!!

I don't know about you folks, but try as I may, over the years, I have NEVER been able to bake french fries or potato wedges... to where I'm actually blissfully happy with them. They are either somewhat floppy and in need of a blue pill... or they are borderline burnt. I combined a tip from America's Test Kitchen, with the addition of cornstarch in the coating. For the first time ever, the clouds parted and the Angels sang in my kitchen.

Ingredients:

- 4 medium russet potatoes. Mine weighed 28oz total.
- Cooking spray
- 1/4 tsp olive oil
- 1/2 tsp salt
- 1/4 tsp pepper
- 1-1/2 tsp garlic powder
- 1/2 tsp smoked paprika
- 1-1/2 tsp cornstarch
- 3 medium cloves garlic, crushed and minced.
- 2 Tbsp fresh parsley, finely chopped, loosely packed.
- *(optional)* 1 tsp reduced fat parmesan topping

Serving Info.:

Yields: 32 wedges
Servings: 4
Serving Size: 8 good sized wedges

Points:

	G	B	P
1 serving =	5	5	0
2 servings =	9	9	0
3 servings =	14	14	0
4 servings =	18	18	0

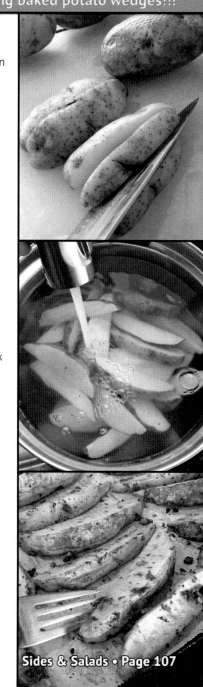

Directions:

1 Preheat oven to 425 degrees. Line a large baking pan with parchment paper, set aside.
2 Slice each potato in half, lengthwise, then slice those halves diagonally, into 4 wedges each.
3 Place the cut wedges into a LARGE bowl, and fill with HOT tap water. Soak potatoes for 10 minutes.
4 Drain wedges, lay them on paper towels, then pat them dry. Set into a large mixing bowl. Spray with a thick 0 point layer of cooking spray, then add 1/4 tsp olive oil. Mix till well coated.
5 In a small bowl, combine the salt, pepper, garlic powder, smoked paprika, cornstarch, garlic, parsley and parmesan (if using).
   Pour over the wedges and mix till coated. Lay the wedges onto the parchment paper lined pan.
6 Bake at 425 degrees for 25 minutes. Remove from oven, then quickly flip all of the wedges. Return to the oven and bake an additional 10-15 minutes, or until brown and crispy. Done.

Notes:

- You should definitely feel free to play around with the seasonings and spices in this recipe. Use my recipe as a stepping stone to make your own flavor combinations.
- If you use jarred garlic, in liquid... this sounds crazy, but scoop the garlic onto a paper towel and pat dry. Otherwise your wedges won't get as crispy, due to the added liquid.
- Honestly... even after 15 minutes out of the oven, these taste like the semi cooled potato wedges that you get at the Jack In The Box drive thru.... with virtually NO FAT.
- I am sooooo jealous of you **PURPLE** Plan people. You must have saint-level restraint around starches.
- At 5 points for Blue folks... this recipe is INSANELY high in points for what I'd normally cook. However, I promised a friend that I'd make actual potato wedges. Besides.... not all of you are as incredibly loco as I am with Point usage. So, you deserve potatoes.

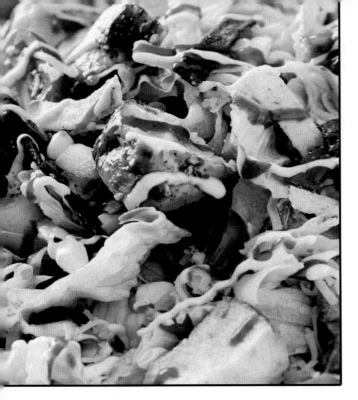

BBQ Ranch Chicken Salad
Ingredients:

- 1/2lb boneless skinless chicken breast, cooked, with salt & pepper, prepared with cooking spray.
- 1/2 cup of my BBQ Sauce, recipe on page 14.
- 1/4 cup of my Ranch dressing, recipe on page 19.
- 4 cups chopped lettuce, any preferred variety.
- 1/2 cup cherry tomatoes, halved
- 1/4 cup reduced fat shredded Mexican style blend cheese (like Kraft)
- 1/2 cup black beans (canned), drained and rinsed
- 1/2 cup whole corn kernels
- 1/4 cup diced red onion
- 1/4 cup chopped fresh cilantro
- (optional) corn tortilla strips, for garnish

Directions:

1 Pre cook the chicken breasts. Saute', grill, grill pan, whatever you want. Chop into chunks, set aside.
2 Prepare the 2 different dressings, in separate bowls. Set aside.
3 In a large bowl, toss together the chicken, lettuce, tomatoes, cheese, black beans, corn, red onion and cilantro. Serve on in a large salad bowl, or in 4 smaller bowls for individual servings.
4 Drizzle 1/2 cup BBQ sauce over the salad(s) and 1/4 cup ranch dressing.
5 (optional) Garnish with corn tortilla strips, or crushed tortilla chips.

Note:

- If you decide to use the corn tortilla strips/bits for garnish, you'll need to add those to the salad points.
- Feel free to add more ranch or more bbq sauce, if desired. However, if you use more than 1/4 cup of my ranch, it will go up 1 point.

Serving Info.:
Servings: 4

Points:	G	B	P
1 serving =	3	1	1
2 servings =	5	2	2
3 servings =	8	2	2
4 servings =	10	3	3

Serving Info.:
Servings: 4

Points:	G	B	P
1 serving =	2	2	2
2 servings =	4	3	3
3 servings =	6	5	5
4 servings =	8	6	6

Blue Cheese Wedge Salad
Ingredients:

- 1/2 batch of my 'Blue Cheese' dressing, recipe found in Cookbook 2, on page 30.
- 1 head of iceberg lettuce, washed, cored, then quartered into 4 wedges.
- 1 slice turkey bacon, cooked till crisp, then crumbled/chopped.
- (optional) diced red pepper, for garnish
- (optional) fresh chives, chopped, for garnish

Directions:

1 Prepare the 1/2 batch of Blue Cheese dressing, set aside. It has a very sharp flavor when first mixed. Allowing it to sit for at least 1 hour makes the flavors mellow and 10x as awesome.
2 Cook the turkey bacon, as much as you can get (brand dependent) for 1 point. Allow it to cool, then chop/crumble it, set aside.
3 Wash and clean 1 head of iceberg lettuce, slice into quarter wedges.
4 Serve by pouring 1/4 cup of dressing over each wedge, sprinkle with crumbled turkey bacon, garnish with optional diced red bell pepper and chives.

Note:

- My recipe takes into account 1 point of turkey bacon. Some brands let you have more than 1 piece for 1 point. Use whatever bacon you wish, but adjust your points if necessary. 1 piece of bacon doesn't sound like much, but once crumbled up, a 1/4 piece can cover a lot of ground.
- Garnish with additional cheese if you wish, but your points will increase.
- If you are making this for a date, I'd recommend serving this salad with breath mints. Ain't nobody getting any action with stinky Blue Cheese breath.

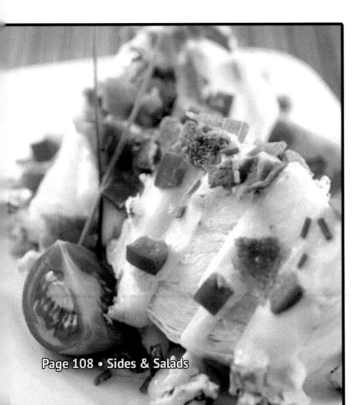

Broccoli Salad

Ingredients:

- 1 slice turkey bacon. Cooked, chopped/crushed.
- 6 cups broccoli florets (1) 12oz bag. Chop any large florets into smaller pieces. We want small-ish florets, not large or even medium sized ones.
- 2 Tbsp shelled sunflower seed kernels, toasted in a hot pan for 2-3 minutes, till fragrant.
- 1/4 cup finely diced red onion
- 2 cups red seeded grapes, sliced in half.

Dressing:
- 1 batch of my 'Creamy Coleslaw Dressing', recipe on pg. 16.

Directions:

1 Cook the turkey bacon till crisp, let it cool, then chop/crumble it. Set aside.
2 Chop any overly large broccoli florets into bite sized pieces.
3 Mix all of the dressing ingredients together, till smooth.
4 Toss all of the ingredients, till well mixed. Cover and rest for 1-2 hours.

Note:

- Some brands of turkey bacon (like Trader Joe's uncured turkey bacon) let you have up to 4 slices for 1 point. My recipe calls for 1 point of bacon. Use more or less if you'd like, but adjust your points per serving accordingly.
- I added my bacon crumbles immediately. Some prefer to add the bacon right before serving, so that it's crunchier. The salad keeps crunch because of the sunflower seeds and diced red onion. I like the added flavor of the bacon, after it sits with the dressing for the 1-2 hours.

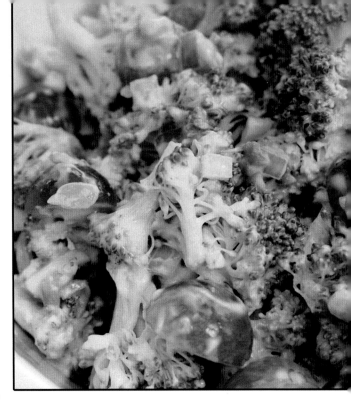

Serving Info.:	Points:	G	B	P
Servings: 7	1 serving =	1	1	1
Serving Size: 1 cup	2 servings =	2	1	1
	3 servings =	3	2	2
	4 servings =	3	3	3

Caesar Salad

Serving Info.:	Points:	G	B	P
Servings: 4	1 serving =	5	3	3
	2 servings =	9	7	7
	3 servings =	14	10	10
	4 servings =	18	13	13

Ingredients:

- 2 slices Sara Lee 45 calorie bread (or other low point bread), cut into crouton sized squares. *(see notes)***
- olive oil cooking spray & dry italian seasonings (for the croutons)
- 1/2 batch of my 'Caesar' dressing, recipe in Cookbook 2, on pg. 32. When preparing the 1/2 batch, make the following changes:
    - Only use 1 egg yolk
    - Only use 1 Tbsp dijon mustard
- 5 cups romaine lettuce, chopped or torn, your preference.
- 2 Tbsp REAL shredded parmesan cheese. I know... go ahead and gasp!
- Fresh cracked black pepper, to taste

Directions:

1 IN ADVANCE: Preheat oven to 350 degrees. Lay the cut bread pieces onto a foil-lined pan. Spray with cooking spray and season with italian seasoning. Flip bread and season other side. Bake the bread slices at 350 degrees for 8-10 minutes, or until croutons are lightly browned and toasted. Set aside.
2 Prepare a 1/2 batch of my Caesar salad dressing, cover, store in the fridge.
3 In a large mixing bowl, toss the romaine with the caesar dressing till well mixed. Add croutons and 1/2 of the parmesan cheese, toss lightly. Top with remaining Parmesan and fresh cracked black pepper. Done.

Note:

- Use whatever low calorie/point bread you want for the croutons. The type that I used is Sara Lee 'delightful' 45 calorie whole wheat bread. 2 slices are 2 points. Adjust your points, depending on the brand you use.
- BLUE & PURPLE folks, to make this a full-on meal, add chicken breast.

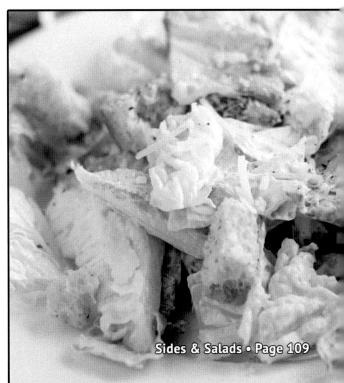

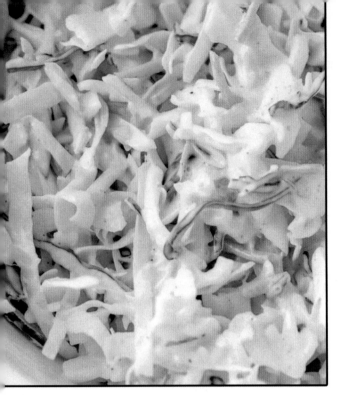

Classic Creamy Coleslaw

Ingredients:

- 16oz bagged coleslaw mix

  Dressing:
- 1/2 cup plain fat free Greek yogurt
- 1 Tbsp light mayonnaise
- 1 Tbsp apple cider vinegar
- 1-1/2 to 2 Tbsp 0 point sweetener o' choice, to taste.
- 1/2 tsp salt
- 1/4 tsp pepper
- (optional) 1 tsp toasted sesame seeds, toast in hot pan for 2-3 minutes.

Directions:

1 Mix all of the dressing ingredients together until thoroughly combined. If using, toast your sesame seeds and add them into the dressing.
2 In a large mixing bowl, combine the coleslaw and dressing till well mixed. The longer it rests, the better it gets.

Note:

- I add the toasted sesame seeds for a little bit of extra flavor and crunch.
- Feel free to add poppy seeds, instead of the sesame seeds, but adjust your points.
- Feel free to use lemon juice instead of apple cider vinegar if you wish.
- You can customize this for Asian slaws, by using rice wine vinegar instead of apple cider. You'd definitely want to go with the sesame seeds then. Maybe even add 1/4 tsp sesame oil for a little extra Asian flavor.

Serving Info.:
Servings: 4

Points:

	G	B	P
1 serving =	1	0	0
2 servings =	1	1	1
3 servings =	2	1	1
4 servings =	2	1	1

Serving Info.:
Servings: 4

Points:

	G	B	P
1 serving =	3	1	1
2 servings =	6	3	3
3 servings =	8	4	4
4 servings =	11	5	5

Cobb Salad

Ingredients:

- 1 batch of my maple mustard dressing, recipe on pg. 18 (see notes)***
- 2 pieces turkey bacon, cooked, chopped/crumbled
- 6 cups romaine lettuce, torn
- 1/2lb chicken breast, cooked, then diced
- 1/2 cup cherry tomatoes
- 2 hard boiled eggs, sliced (good luck, I suck at not mutilating them).
- 1/4 cup reduced fat shredded cheese (see notes)***
- 1/2 small red onion, thin sliced
- 1/2 cup peas

Directions:

1 In a large bowl, combine the dressing, lettuce, chicken, tomatoes, shredded cheese, red onion and peas. Mix till well combined.
2 Serve in a large salad bowl, or in 4 smaller individual bowls.
3 Arrange the hardboiled egg and crumbled/chopped turkey bacon among the 4 servings, or onto the large salad bowl.

Note:

- I used my maple mustard (my version of honey mustard) dressing on my Cobb salad, because that's my personal preference. However, I encourage you to use WHATEVER dressing you want. My 2nd favorite for a Cobb, of my dressings, is the 'Apple Vinaigrette' in Cookbook 2.
- You can slice the cherry tomatoes in half, if you prefer.
- It's more traditional to chop the hardboiled eggs, rather than slicing them.
- Instead of mixing everything together with the dressing, you can serve it as pictured. Mix the salad ingredients together, but serve the dressing on the side.
- I used 2 points of turkey bacon. Feel free to use whatever brand or type of bacon you want, but adjust points if necessary.

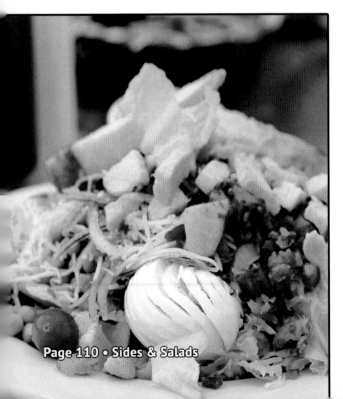

Creamy Roasted Garlic & Onion Pasta

Ingredients:

- 6 oz dried macaroni, shells, or other small pasta.
  I used "ditalini" pasta (pictured to the right)
- 1/2 to 3/4 cup of my 'Roasted Garlic & Onion' dressing, recipe in my
  Cookbook Volume 2, on pg. 34. *(points stay the same at 1/2 or 3/4c)*
- 2 medium zucchini, sliced into bite sized pieces.
- 2 medium yellow squash, cut into bite sized pieces.
- 1 medium red onion, diced.
- 6 oz fresh broccoli florets.
- 1/2 cup whole corn kernels
- salt and pepper to taste
- 1/2 cup fresh basil, chopped

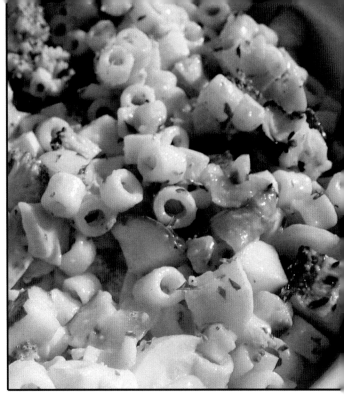

Directions:

1. Prepare the salad dressing, set aside.
2. Cook the pasta according to box directions, drain, set aside.
3. Place broccoli florets into gallon sized ziplock bag with 1 Tbsp water. Close the bag, poke a small hole in it with a knife, then microwave for 2 minutes. Remove to cutting board, chop into bite sized pieces. Set aside.
4. Heat a large pan over medium-high heat for 1 minute. Spray with cooking spray and add the onion, zucchini, yellow squash and corn. Season with salt and pepper, cook over medium-high heat for 6-7 minutes. Set aside.
5. In a large mixing bowl, combine all of the ingredients, including the fresh chopped basil. Mix to combine. Season with salt and pepper to taste.

Note:

- This pasta salad is even better if you grill your vegetables, then chop them up, rather than cook them in a pan.

Serving Info.:
Servings: 6
Serving Size: 1 cup

Points:	G	B	P
1 serving =	4	3	3
2 servings =	8	6	6
3 servings =	12	9	9
4 servings =	16	12	12

Crunchy Asian Chicken Salad

Serving Info.:
Servings: 4

Points:	G	B	P
1 serving =	2	1	1
2 servings =	3	2	2
3 servings =	5	3	3
4 servings =	6	4	4

Ingredients:

- 1/2lb chicken breast, cooked, chopped, set aside.
- 1 batch of my rice wine dressing, recipe on pg. 19, with the following additions:
  * Add 1 more Tbsp vinegar. * Add 2 more tsp sweetener.
  * Include the optional toasted sesame seeds
- 4 cups chopped romaine lettuce
- 4 green onions, thin sliced (just the green parts)
- Small can of mandarin oranges, drained and rinsed
- 1/4 package dry ramen noodles (just the dried noodles, no seasoning)
- 1 Tbsp roasted pumpkin seed kernels

Directions:

1. Cook the chicken, chop, set aside. Prepare a batch of the salad dressing with the listed modifications, set aside.
2. Open a can of mandarin oranges, drain and rinse off the oranges, set aside. Then open a package of ramen noodles, break off 1/4 of the noodles, crush and set aside.
3. In a large mixing bowl, combine ALL of the ingredients together until thoroughly mixed. Allow to rest for 10 minutes before serving.

Note:

- Buy a small can of mandarin oranges, drain and rinse them, then use as many of the small orange segments as you'd personally like.
- We're only using 1/4 of a package of dried ramen noodles, they are really high in points, and even the small amount really adds a great crunch to the salad.

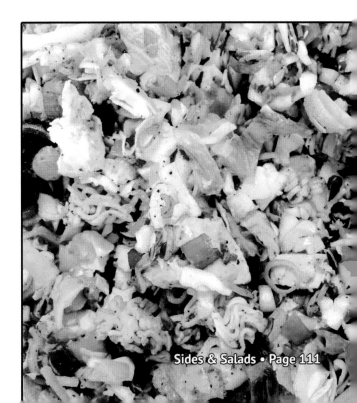

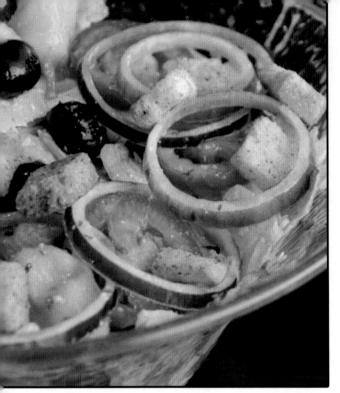

Mediterranean Salad *(Olive Garden copycat)*
Ingredients:

- 2 slices Sara Lee 45 calorie bread (or other low point bread), cut into crouton sized squares. *(see notes)***
- Italian seasoning (for croutons)
- 1 batch of my Creamy Italian Dressing, recipe on pg. 18
- 6 cups romaine lettuce, chopped or torn, your preference.
- 8 canned black olives, pitted (you can slice them if you want, I didn't).
- 1/2 small red onion, sliced into thin rings
- 6 mild pepperoncini peppers (found near the jarred pickles and olives).
- 2 roma tomatoes, sliced into 1/4" thick rounds.
- 1 Tbsp grated parmesan cheese... the REAL stuff. *gasp*
- Fresh cracked black pepper, to taste

Directions:

1. <u>IN ADVANCE:</u> Preheat oven to 350 degrees. Lay the cut bread pieces onto a foil-lined pan. Spray with cooking spray and season with italian seasoning. Flip bread and season other side. Bake the bread slices at 350 degrees for 8-10 minutes, or until croutons are lightly browned and toasted. Set aside.
2. In a large mixing bowl, combine the lettuce, olives, red onion slices, pepperoncini peppers and sliced tomatoes.
3. Add the dressing and croutons, toss to combine. Top with Parmesan cheese and fresh cracked black pepper, to taste.

Note:

- 8 whole black olives isn't a lot, so if you'd like more bang for your buck, slice the olives, so they spread throughout the salad.
- Use whatever low calorie/low point bread you want for the croutons. The type that I used is Sara Lee 'delightful' 45 calorie whole wheat bread. 2 slices are 2 points. Adjust your points, depending on the brand you use.

Serving Info.:	Points:		G	B	P
Servings: 4	1 serving =		1	1	1
	2 servings =		2	2	2
	3 servings =		4	2	2
	4 servings =		5	3	3

Serving Info.:	Points:		G	B	P
Servings: 5	1 serving =		6	1	1
Size: 3/4 cup	2 servings =		13	1	1
	3 servings =		19	2	2
	4 servings =		26	2	2

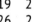

Mexican 'Street Corn' Salad
Ingredients:

- 6 cups fresh corn kernels or (2) 15oz cans of whole kernel corn, drained.
- 2 medium garlic cloves, crushed and chopped
- butter flavored cooking spray
- 1/2 tsp salt
- 1/4 tsp pepper
- 1/2 cup plain fat free Greek yogurt
- 1 Tbsp light mayonnaise
- 2 Tbsp lime juice
- 1/2 cup diced red onion
- 1/2 cup chopped fresh cilantro, loosely packed
- 1/4 cup green onion, thin slice, loosely packed
- 1/4 cup reduced fat feta cheese crumbles *(you can use 'fat free', adjust points)*.
- a dusting of chili powder or paprika, to taste, for garnish (**SEE NOTES**)***

Directions:

1. Drain the canned corn kernels, spread onto paper towels, pat dry.
2. Heat a large pan over medium-high heat for 1 minute, then spray with butter flavored cooking spray. Add corn, garlic, salt and pepper. Cook on medium-high heat for 10-15 minutes, allowing the corn to sit still for 1-2 minutes at a time. You want to start getting a slight 'char' to the corn. Once the corn is covered with light black char marks, pour it into a large mixing bowl with the red and green onion, feta cheese and chopped cilantro. Toss to combine.
3. Stir together the yogurt, mayo and lime juice, then mix into the salad. Done.

Note:

- You can definitely cook ears of corn on the grill for this, till they are lightly charred. I used a pan for this recipe, because not everyone owns a grill.
- When serving, garnish with a dusting of chili powder OR paprika. The chili powder definitely makes it a little spicy. If you don't like heat, use paprika.

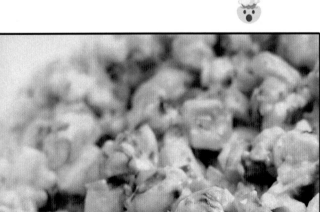

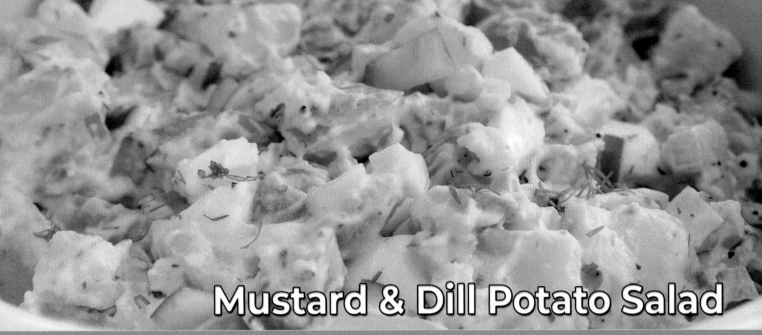

Mustard & Dill Potato Salad

A Lightened Up, Snazzy Potato Salad, Customizable To Your Liking

This is my lightened up version of Ina Garten's famous potato salad. Like most 'famous' recipes online, the original was loaded with enough full fat mayonnaise to send Fat Albert to his cardiologist. Anyone can make food taste good if it's loaded with butter, mayo and bacon grease. In this lightened version, we're cutting fat free Greek yogurt with a touch of light mayo. Next, we're thinning it with a little water and some dill pickle relish for added zing. All in all, we end up cutting about 50 billion calories from a regular recipe, but what's new.

Ingredients:

- 1.5 pounds of <u>small</u> yellow potatoes. You can use any <u>thin skinned</u>, small potato variety you like. If you use large potatoes, increase the boiling time.
- 1/2 cup fat free plain Greek yogurt
- 1 Tbsp light mayonnaise
- 1 Tbsp dijon mustard
- 1 Tbsp stone ground mustard (*see notes*)***
- 1 Tbsp water
- 2-3 Tbsp dill pickle relish, to taste.
- 3-4 Tbsp fresh dill, finely chopped, to taste.
- 1-/2 to 3/4 tsp salt, to taste.
- 1/2 tsp pepper
- 1/3 cup diced red onion
- 1/2 cup diced celery
- 2 large hardboiled eggs, chop the egg whites, discard yolks. (*see notes*)***

Serving Info.:

Yields: 5-1/2 cups
Servings: 7
Serving Size: 3/4 cup

Points:

	G	B	P
1 serving =	2	2	0
2 servings =	5	4	0
3 servings =	7	6	0
4 servings =	9	9	1

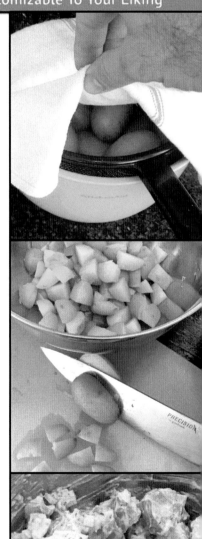

Directions:

1 Bring a pot of water to a boil over medium-high heat. Add potatoes and boil for 15 minutes. Drain water, keep the potatoes in a strainer and cover with a towel. Allow to cool, covered, for 10 minutes.

2 While the potatoes are resting, covered, Mix together the yogurt, mayo, 2 mustards, water, relish, fresh dill, salt and pepper, till well combined. Set aside.

3 After the potatoes have rested for 15 minutes, move them to a cutting board and slice into bite sized pieces. Make them as large or as small as you wish. I personally cut the medium sized potatoes into 1/8's and the smaller potatoes into 1/4's.

4 In a large mixing bowl, gently fold together the potatoes with the dill dressing. When well mixed, fold in the diced red onions and celery. Lastly, fold in the chopped egg whites. Cover and let sit in the fridge for 20-30 minutes, then taste and season with additional salt and pepper or relish, to taste. Done.

Note:

- GREENIES: We're using 2 chopped up egg whites, rather than whole eggs, to save you a point. If you're on **BLUE** or **PURPLE**, feel free to add as many chopped up eggs as'ya want.
- '*Stone Ground Mustard*': Different brands of stone ground mustard allow you to have different amounts for 0 points. Scan the brands at your store. "Organics" stone ground mustard lets you have 1 Tbsp for 0. Most brands only let you have 2 tsp. Use whatever brand you can, but use a 0 point amount of what's available.
- **Fresh Dill**: If you don't like dill, try subbing it with chives. This is a very customizable recipe.
- The <u>original</u> recipe is 11 points per serving. It also has an extra 1,961 calories and 165 grams more fat.

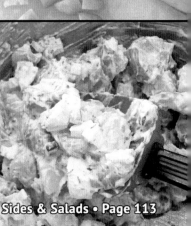

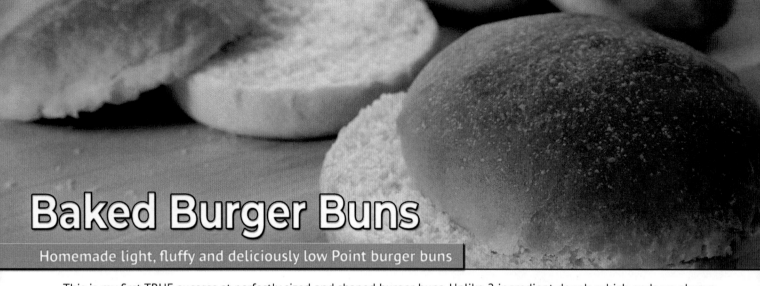

Baked Burger Buns

Homemade light, fluffy and deliciously low Point burger buns

This is my first TRUE success at perfectly sized and shaped burger buns. Unlike 2 ingredient dough, which ends up always tasting like a biscuit, these buns have a great texture, brown beautifully, taste like REAL BREAD and have a soft, light and fluffy interior. I know that a lot of us can buy 2-3 point burger buns at our local stores, but not everyone has access to those, so these are a great option. Plus, they are homemade, so you know exactly what is in them... and what's in them is delicious.

			G	B	P
Servings Info.:	**Points:**	1 serving =	3	3	3
Yield: 4 buns		2 servings =	7	7	7
Serving Size: 1 bun		3 servings =	10	10	10
		4 servings =	13	13	13

Ingredients:

- 3 tsp active dry yeast
- 2-1/4 tsp granulated sugar (you can't use sweetener)
- 1/2 cup water (<u>MUST</u> be between 100-110 degrees)
- 3/4 cup PLUS 1-1/2 tsp all purpose flour. To make that easy, measure 1 cup of flour, then <u>remove</u> 1-1/2 Tbsp. Easy.
- Cooking Spray, flavored (butter, olive oil, whatever you want).
- 1/4 tsp olive, canola or vegetable oil
- 1/4 tsp salt
- additional water, only if necessary (1 tsp at a time)

Directions:

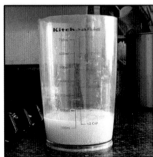 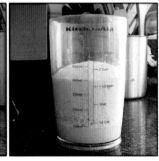

1. Scoop the active dry yeast and sugar into a tall container or cup. I know it sounds food-snooty, but it's VERY important... stir in 1/2 cup of 100-110 degree water. Use a thermometer if you have one, you <u>need</u> it to be between 100-110 degrees. Stir the water gently till mixed, then allow to sit, untouched, for 15 minutes.

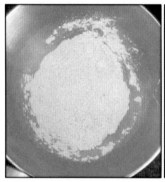 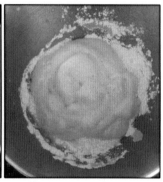

2. While the yeast is rising, Turn on your oven so that it preheats to 425 degrees. While it's heating up and your yeast is 'blooming', add the flour, salt and 1/4 tsp oil to a large mixing bowl. Spray into the bowl for 6 to 8 seconds (0 point amount, per your brand) of cooking spray. Then after the yeast has 'bloomed' for 15 minutes, pour the yeast-liquid into the bowl.

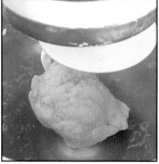 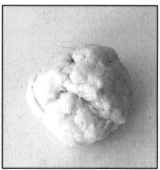

3. Begin mixing the dry and wet ingredients together. The mixture will be a bit wet, but that's ok. Use a rubber spatula to scrape down the sides and continue mixing. It will have the consistency of very thick brownie batter at this point. Just trust me.. If it's a little tacky, don't worry about it. Spritz a cutting board with a light mist of cooking spray then scoop the soft dough onto it. The dough will still be pretty wet. It's ok.

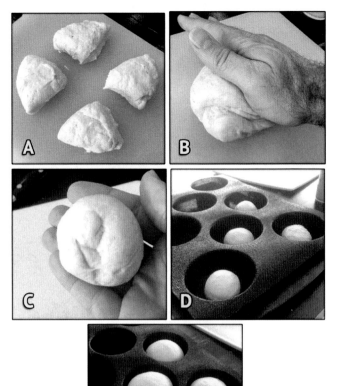

- <u>FORGOT TO MENTION!!!</u> I purchased an inexpensive rubber silicone "hamburger bun mold" on Amazon, to use for this recipe. This way, the dough forms, and bakes into a perfect hamburger bun shape. Get one with small perforations all around the cavities. Set the mold on a baking tray to use it.
- If you are allergic to gluten, you can make this recipe with gluten free flour. Bob's Red Mill has a really good Gluten Free '**1 to 1 Baking Flour**', that's available in many major supermarkets. Make sure to adjust your points, if necessary..
- You can use this recipe as a base and add your own flair to it. Add onions, garlic, cheddar cheese, sesame seeds, etc.
- If you don't have a mold, you can set the dough balls onto a baking pan and let them rise. However, it is a 'loose' dough. It won't take on the perfect shape of a burger bun, but that's ok. You're here to eat, not to make googly eyes at your buns... unless you're into that sorta thing. I won't judge.
- Double this recipe and rather than section it for buns, season the dough and use it for breadsticks. Look online for suggestions for cooking times with similar baked goods.
- Though these buns are tasty and delicious... they are NOT as large as regular store bought buns. Primarily because this recipe is using less flour than traditional recipes, due to my attempts at making a 'low point' bun, that's Weight Watchers compliant. If you are not on Weight Watchers, or don't care about 'Points', use 1-1/4 cup flour. The buns will bake up much taller.

4. The dough will be pretty tacky and difficult to form, just spray it with a little cooking spray. It helps a lot.
   (A) Cut the ball into 4 equal sections, then **(B)** Gently fold each ball over itself about 15-20 times. **(C)** Roll the dough into a small ball in your palm. It will still be very very soft, that's what we want. **(D)** Place the seam side down, in the silicone mold, spray the top with cooking spray, then **(E)** walk away for 15 minutes. NO TOUCHING!

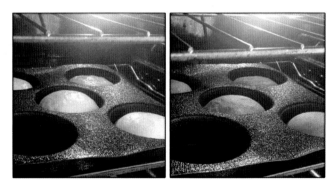

5. Bake the buns for 12-14 minutes, depending on how golden brown you want them to look. Remove from the oven, then.... trust me on this... put them in a bowl and cover it, or put them in a gallon sized ziplock bag. Let them 'steam', covered, for 5 minutes. It softens them and they take on a pillow softness. Right out of the oven they will have a hard crust, but resting, covered, will soften them up.

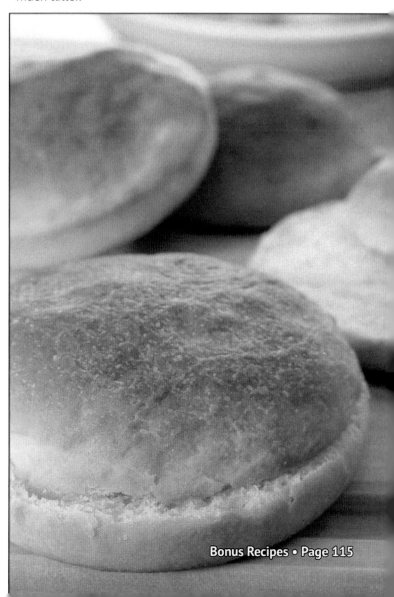

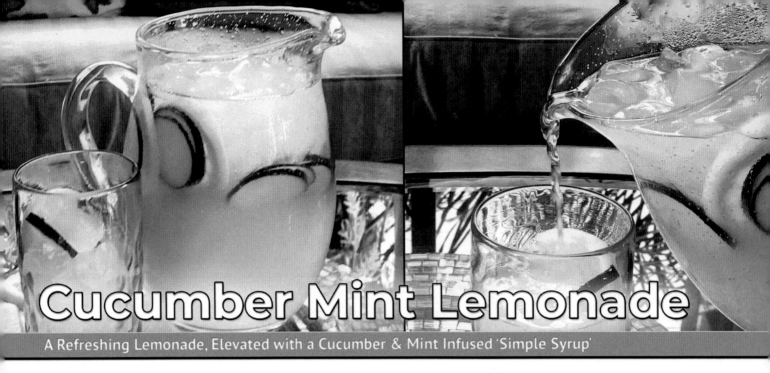

Cucumber Mint Lemonade

A Refreshing Lemonade, Elevated with a Cucumber & Mint Infused 'Simple Syrup'

Years ago, back when I was still fat-Dan, I worked at a machine shop as a Lathe Operator. One day, the owner took me to a local Mexican restaurant where they had the most amazing lemonade. It took 6 months before we got the recipe out of the owner. The regular recipe uses a butt-load of sugar and a spoonful of honey. My skinnied version uses 0 calorie sweetener and sugar free syrup. So that we don't have grainy sugar at the bottom of our lemonade, we're making a steeped 'simple syrup', by simmering some cucumber slices, lemon juice, sweetener, water and fresh mint. **NOTE:** The listed points are with Lakanto monkfruit. You can use any '0 calorie' sugar substitute you wish, but adjust your points.

Servings Info.:

Yields: 8 cups (2 quarts)
Servings: 8
Serving Size: 8oz (1 cup)

Points:

	G	B	P
1 serving =	0	0	0
2 servings =	0	0	0
3 servings =	0	0	0
4 servings =	1	1	1

Ingredients:

Not So Simple Syrup

- 3/4 cup 0 point sweetener (I used Lakanto Monkfruit)
- 3/4 cups lemon juice (I used bottled)
- 1 cup water
- 1 Tbsp sugar free syrup (pancake syrup)
- 1 sprig fresh mint
- 1/2 large cucumber, sliced into thin rounds
- dash of salt

Additional Ingredients:

- 1/2 cucumber (the leftover, unused half, from the syrup)
- 1 lemon, thin sliced, around 1/4" thick, remove seeds
- 2-3 sprigs fresh mint, attached to the center stem
- 6 cups Cold Water, and/or Ice, in any combination. Whether you use more water, or more ice, try to use 6-1/2 cups worth. If you add ALL water, then add ice, it'll water down your lemonade's flavor.

Directions:

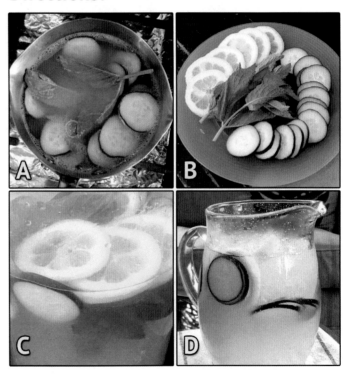

1. **(A)** Bring all of the 'simple syrup' ingredients to a low boil in a small pot, for 3 minutes. Remove from heat and set aside, allowing the syrup to cool for 20 minutes. **(B)** Slice the remaining half of the cucumber, into thin rounds. Slice half of the lemon into rounds, removing any seeds. Lastly, wash 2-3 sprigs of fresh mint, set aside. **(C)** Remove and discard the wilted cucumber and mint from the syrup. Pour the cooled syrup into a large 2 quart pitcher with the the 6-1/2 cups of cold water/ice. Add the fresh mint and cucumber/lemon slices. Set in the fridge to continue cooling. **(D)** You can serve in the 2 quart pitcher, or serve in a 1 quart pitcher, giving you extra to keep in the fridge, for refills.

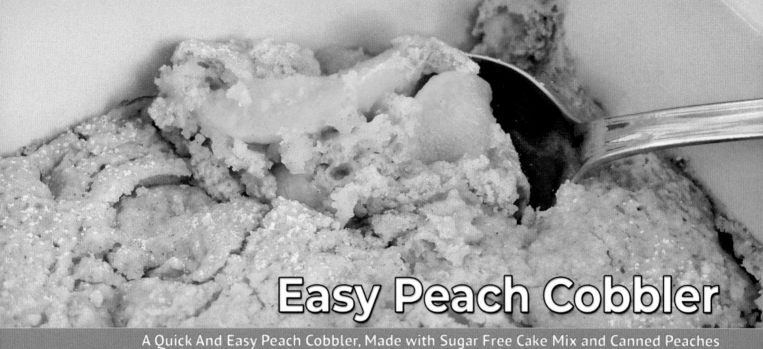

Easy Peach Cobbler

A Quick And Easy Peach Cobbler, Made with Sugar Free Cake Mix and Canned Peaches

When my wife's family used to get together (back when family get togethers were still legal... 😷 there was one dessert that I ALWAYS looked forward to. My Brother In Law's Peach Cobbler. He's a Fire Captain, has to cook for macho men, so as you can imagine, his cobbler is legit. When I was finalizing this book, I realized that I didn't really have any desserts in it. I figured it'd be nice to have an easy peach cobbler recipe that folks could make, but it HAD to be low in calories and fat. Easiest way to accomplish that? Use sugar free yellow cake mix as the base. You can also use fresh peaches, but I prefer canned peaches in a cobbler. I prefer the softer texture.

Ingredients:

- 1 Pillsbury sugar free 'supreme' yellow cake mix
- 1/2 tsp ground cinnamon
- 2 Tbsp 0 point natural sweetener o' choice
- (3) 15oz cans sliced peaches, in water (or no sugar added), drained and rinsed, to ensure 0 points.
- 1-1/4 cup water
- Butter flavored cooking spray
- 13x9 baking pan or casserole
- (optional) 1/2 tsp powdered sugar, to dust, for garnish.

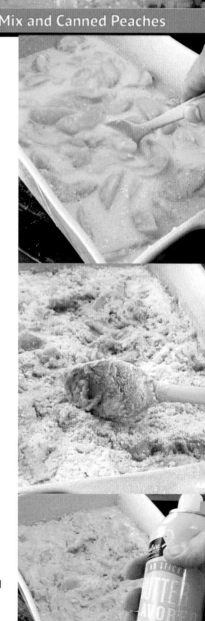

Serving Info.:

Yields: (1) 13"x9" casserole pan
Servings: 12
Serving Size: 2/3 cup

Points:

	G	B	P
1 serving =	3	3	3
2 servings =	6	6	6
3 servings =	10	10	10
4 servings =	13	13	13

Directions:

1 Preheat oven to 350 degrees. Lightly spray 13x9 baking dish with cooking spray, set side.
2 In a large bowl, mix together the cake mix, cinnamon and sweetener.
3 Add HALF of the mixed dry ingredients into the bottom of the baking dish. Pour the rinsed and drained sliced peaches over the dry ingredients, followed by the water. Gently stir to combine.
4 Pour the remaining dry ingredients over the top of the 'battered' peach slices, then stir till mostly mixed in.
5 Coat the top of the batter with a good 0 point amount of butter flavored cooking spray.
6 Bake at 350 degrees for 40-45 minutes, or until an inserted toothpick comes out mostly clean. You want it to have just a tiny bit of moist crumb still, on the bottom of the toothpick. You don't want a fully set cake. You want this to be a still-moist cross between a cake and a cobbler.
7 (optional) When the cake comes out of the oven, put 1/2 tsp powdered sugar into a fine wire mess strainer. Lightly tap the strainer while holding it over the cake, to lightly dust it.

Note:

- You can find a ton of variations of this type of easy cake, online. They are traditionally called a 'dump cake'. But because the name 'Dump Cake' is a COMPLETELY UNAPPEALING term for food... yeah. I'm not calling mine that. Regardless, use mine as a template. It's pretty easy to lower the calories and fat in any of them, with a few smart ingredients swaps.
- Want a cool idea for a chocolate version? Use a Pillsbury sugar free devil's food cake mix. Instead of canned peaches, add a few cups of fresh dark cherries, plus the water. Add some rum extract... Hellooooo, nurse.
- Butter Flavored Cooking Spray?!?!: Yup, trust me. Scan your can to see how much you can use to stay at 0 points. I was able to use a solid 8 second buttery spray. It gave a great butter flavor to the dish. The regular recipes call for an entire 1/2 stick of butter, melted and poured onto the top of the cobbler. That's because regular food bloggers and 'celebrity' chefs don't care if you gain weight from eating their food. I do.

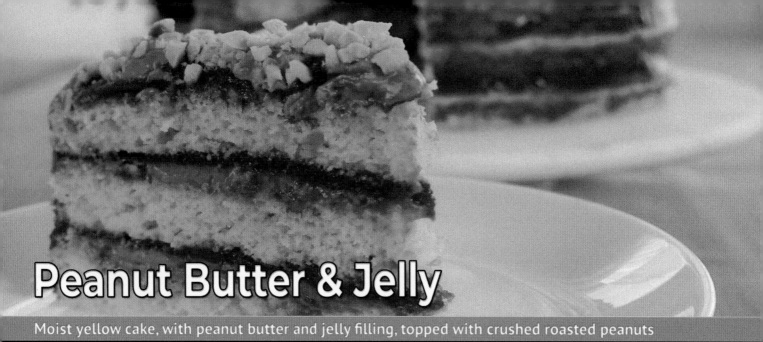

Peanut Butter & Jelly

Moist yellow cake, with peanut butter and jelly filling, topped with crushed roasted peanuts

I absolutely love PB&J. Yes, if you are a 7 year old and want to ask... Yeah, I'd marry it. That being said, after making this cake earlier today, this is now my absolute favorite cake. This is a fancy 3 layered cake version of my cupcake recipe, don't want to go all super fancy? No worries, there are notes for making a simpler 2 layer version.

Ingredients:

Cake Batter:
- 1 sugar free yellow cake mix
- 1 egg
- 1-1/3 cup club soda, seltzer water or any 0 point carbonated beverage.
- 1 tsp baking powder

Strawberry Jelly Filling:
- 4 cups strawberries, fresh or frozen. I used 2 (10oz) bags of frozen whole strawberries.
- 1/4 cup water
- 1 (0.6oz) box sugar free strawberry flavored gelatin. *(You can use raspberry gelatin if you can't find strawberry)*
- 1/4 cup 0 point sweetener of choice (splenda, swerve, monkfruit, truvia, stevia, etc.)
- 1/2 tsp strawberry extract *(in the baking aisle, by the vanilla)*
- 1/4 cup + 2 tsp cornstarch, dissolved in 1/4 cup additional water.
- 1 tsp lemon juice

Peanut Butter & Butterscotch Pudding
- 2 (1oz) boxes Jello sugar free, instant butterscotch pudding
- 1-1/4 cup powdered peanut butter
- 1/8 tsp salt
- 1-3/4 cups cold water

Topping
- 1/3 cup salted roasted peanuts, measured, then crushed.

Serving Info.:
YIELDS: 12 slices
Servings: 12
Serving Size: 1/12 slice

Points:

	G	B	P
1 serving =	7	6	6
2 servings =	12	12	12
3 servings =	19	18	18
4 servings =	25	24	24

Directions:

1 Preheat oven to 325.
2 Line the bottom of (3) 9 inch round pans with parchment paper. Spray the sides of the pans with cooking spray. Set aside.

*** CAKE DIRECTIONS
3 In a large mixing bowl, combine the cake mix, egg, baking powder and carbonated beverage o' choice. Mix to combine.
4 Use a 1/2 cup measuring scoop, to pour an equal amount of batter into each of the 3 pans. It SHOULD be just over 1-1/2 cups of batter in each pan.
5 Bake at 325 for 20-24 minutes, or until a toothpick inserted into the center comes out clean. Cooking times may vary depending on your oven, altitude... or attitude.
6 When the toothpick comes out dry, remove the cakes from the oven and allow to cool in the pans. Set aside.

*** STRAWBERRY JELLY FILLING
7 Add the strawberries, 1/4 cup water, powdered gelatin, sweetener o' choice and strawberry extract to a medium sized pot. Stir the ingredients, cover and bring to a simmer for 3-4 minutes, until the strawberries are softened.
8 Use a blender, or an immersion blender, to puree everything together until smooth.
9 Bring it back to a simmer, then add the dissolved cornstarch. Stir until well combined. Simmer the puree, uncovered, for 4-5 minutes, stirring occasionally.
10 Pour the puree into a large heat resistant dish or mixing bowl. Cover with plastic wrap, allow it to cool down for a few hours, moving it into the fridge until set.

*** BUTTERSCOTCH & PEANUT BUTTER PUDDING

11 In a mixing bowl (I personally like using an empty 32oz Greek yogurt container for this), add the dry pudding, powdered peanut butter, salt and cold water.

12 Use an electric hand mixer to mix the ingredients until thick and smooth. Set aside in the fridge.

*** TOPPING DIRECTIONS

13 Fill a 1/3 cup measuring scoop with dry roasted peanuts. Pour the peanuts into a ziplock bag, then grab a kitchen mallet, a phone book, or a typical receipt from CVS Pharmacy and beat the ever-loving snot out of those peanuts. Go full-blown whack-a-mole on them.

14 Place the crushed bits of peanut destruction into a small bowl, set them aside for later.

*** ASSEMBLY

15 Take one of your cake layers and spread a thin layer of peanut butter pudding, about 1/4 inch, across it from edge to edge. Then spread an equal amount of the cooled jelly on top of the peanut butter, from edge to edge.

16 Place the 2nd cake layer on top, then repeat the process for the 2nd layer. Cake, peanut butter, then strawberry jelly.

17 Now, we switch it up. For the TOP layer.... place the top layer of cake down, but this time, spread the jelly first, THEN top that with peanut butter. Trust me.

18 Take your crushed peanuts and sprinkle them all over the top of the cake, from edge to edge, as best as you can. The finer that you crush them, the more coverage you'll get.

19 If you want, you can take some of your remaining strawberry jelly, like I did, and use a rubber spatula to smear a thin layer around the outside of the cake. It will help keep the cake from drying out. It IS an optional step though. You can leave the cake "naked" on the sides if you prefer that look.

20 Apologize to your guests that are allergic to peanuts.

*** NOTES

-   If you are allergic to peanuts, but not to almonds, many grocery stores now sell powdered almond butter, rather than ONLY selling powdered peanut butter. Use that, along with crushed almonds on top.

-   If you don't want strawberry jelly, feel free to use Jello sugar free raspberry or black cherry gelatin instead. Then, you'd obviously swap out the fruit as well.

-   If you'd like to, you could definitely go the simpler route and make a regular 2 layered cake, rather than a 3 layered cake like I did. Simply divide the cake batter into 2 pans instead of 3. The baking time will increase to 30-35 minutes. You will also want to use a much thicker layer of the peanut butter and jelly for the filling, as well as for frosting the top of the cake. Keep the side frosting thin, or it could possibly run down the side of your cake if too heavy.

-   If you are allergic to gluten, Swerve makes a sugar free, gluten free cake mix. I haven't personally used it, and I'm not sure what the points are for it, but you can look into it as an option. Worst case, a regular cake mix will only raise the point value for this cake by 2-3 points for 1 slice.

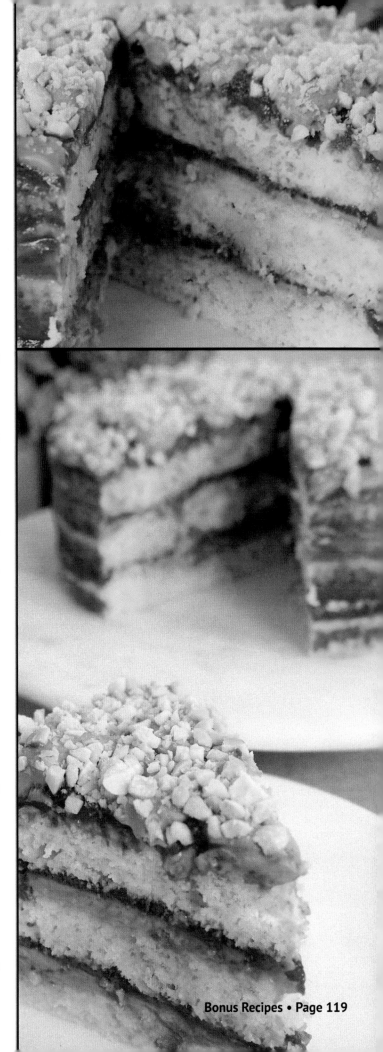

Personal Mini Cake

A Delicious, Fast & Highly Customizable Mini Cocoa Cake

Unlike all of my other cake and cupcake recipes, which are based on the use of Pillsbury sugar free cake mixes, I wanted to make a small, low point, single serving cake that could be made with a few simple ingredients. There are a lot of people that are sheltered in their houses right now, unable to get typical ingredients. This small cake is meant to be made by people who have to ration what they have during all these 'bleepity-bleepin' stay at home orders.

This is a low calorie take on a personal sized "*Depression Cake*", which is a cake recipe made popular during the Great Depression, when ingredients were scarce and rationed. Typical recipes for this type of cake call for a lot of oil and sugar. I'm lowering the calories by replacing the oil with water and the sugar with natural 0 point sweetener.

Ingredients:

- 4 Tbsp + 1 tsp all purpose flour **
- 1/4 tsp baking soda
- 1/8 tsp baking powder
- pinch of salt
- 1 Tbsp unsweetened cocoa powder
- 2-1/2 Tbsp 0 point sweetener o' choice**
  (*monkfruit, swerve, stevia, splenda, etc.*), adjust to your tastes.
- 1 tsp vanilla extract
- 2 tsp vinegar**
- 4 Tbsp water
- 1/4 tsp powdered sugar, for garnish.

Serving Info.:

Yields: 1 mini cake
Servings: 1
Serving Size: 1 cake

Points: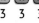

1 serving =   3   3   3

Directions:

1 Preheat oven to 375 degrees. In two separate bowls, prepare the dry and wet ingredients, separately.
2 Quickly mix all the ingredients into a batter, then pour into an 8oz ramekin, sprayed with cooking spray. ONLY fill the ramekin 3/4 full, it's ok if there is a tiny bit of batter left over. Don't overfill the ramekin or the cake will spill out over the sides while baking.
3 Bake at 375 degrees for 20 minutes.
4 If you'd like to "snazzy it up", use a wire mesh strainer, to dust the top of the mini cake with powdered sugar. Done.

Note:

- If you do not want to use 0 point sugar substitute, obviously..... use regular sugar, but adjust your points. And MAKE SURE to use a sweetener that is FOR BAKING!!!! The package will say how much to substitute for sugar in recipes.
- You can use any flour that you have on hand for this recipe, though each will give a slightly different finished texture. I used all purpose flour for mine. If you are allergic to Gluten, feel free to try this recipe with gluten free flour, such as Bob's Red Mill.
- I used 8oz ramekins. Don't have a ramekin? Use a cupcake/muffin pan, it should work, but will look like a mushroom cloud.
- Use any type of vinegar that you have on hand, even balsamic. At only 2 teaspoons, most all vinegars stay 0 points.
- The powdered sugar is for dusting. If you are on a sugar free diet, use "Swerve" or Lakanto brand, 0 point powdered sugar substitute.
- **IMPORTANT NOTE!!**: Any brand Stevia with Maltodystrine can have an off-putting taste when used in recipes with vinegar. If your stevia has that ingredient as a filler... don't use it. Also... "Monkfruit In The Raw" brand sweetener tastes absolutely disgusting.
- This recipe is for 1 single mini cake. You can easily double, triple, or quadruple the batter. Mix it all as a large batch, then quickly pour into multiple ramekins.

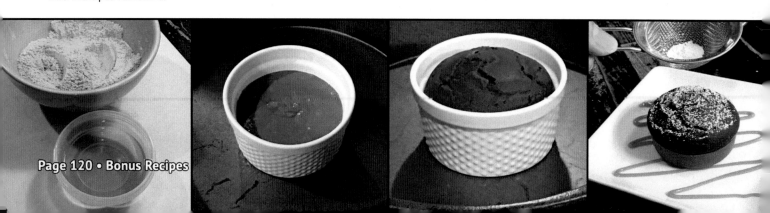

Almond Cake:

Recipe Changes:

- Remove the cocoa powder.
- Replace the vanilla extract with almond extract, found in the baking/spice aisle.
- Add 2 tsp powdered peanut butter or powdered almond butter.
- Add 1/8 tsp ground cinnamon (helps with color). Measure a 0 point amount of almonds, by weight, then crush them. Sprinkle the crushed almonds on top of the cake batter, right before baking. Don't have almonds? Use crushed walnuts instead, but weigh them and check points.

Blueberry Cake:

Recipe Changes:

- Remove the cocoa powder.
- Use any vinegar other than balsamic.
- Replace all the water with 1/4 cup pureed blueberries.
- Increase bake time by 5-10 minutes. Insert toothpick.

Carrot Cake:

Recipe Changes:

- Remove the cocoa powder.
- Add 1/4 tsp ground cinnamon.
- Add 1/8 tsp ground nutmeg.
- Add EITHER 1/4 tsp of molasses into the wet ingredients, or replace the 0 point sweetener with 0 point brown sugar substitute... It's your choice.
- Finely chop up a few baby carrots, and add 3 Tbsp of the carrots into the dry ingredients.
- Measure a 0 point amount of walnuts, by weight, then crush them and add into the dry ingredients. I was able to get 1 tsp of loosely packed, crushed walnuts.
- (optional) measure a 0 point amount of raisins, by weight, if you'd like to have them in your carrot cake.
- Bake for 25-30 minutes, or 'til a toothpick comes out clean.

Hummingbird Cake: (banana & pineapple)

Recipe Changes:

- Remove the cocoa powder.
- Add 1/8 tsp ground cinnamon.
- ONLY use 2 Tbsp of sweetener
- Instead of using the 1/4 cup of water, in the base recipe... Open a can of crushed pineapple. Rinse and drain it, so that it's 0 points. Add 3 Tbsp crushed, rinsed pineapple into the wet ingredients, in place of the water.
- Mash half of a banana with some water, till it's a smooth and pureed consistency. Add 2 Tbsp of the banana "puree" to the wet ingredients.
- Replace the vanilla extract with maple extract. If your batter is too thick, add 1 Tbsp water, while mixing.
- Bake for 25-30 mins., until a toothpick comes out clean.

Flavor Variations

By modifying the "base" cake recipe, from the previous page, you can make a wide variety of snazzy mini cakes. The following flavored cakes are made by slightly modifying the base-cake recipe with different extracts and spices. You can also find 13 additional flavors on my website, in the 'desserts' link, under 'Quarantine Mini Cake'.

Lemon Cake:

Recipe Changes:

- Remove the cocoa powder.
- Leave out the vinegar from the recipe.
- Replace the vanilla extract with lemon extract, found in the baking/spice aisle.
- Replace 3 Tbsp of the water with 3 Tbsp of lemon juice.
- Add 1 additional Tbsp water, if the batter is too thick.

Peanut Butter Chocolate Cake:

Recipe Changes:

- Add 2 tsp powdered peanut butter.
- Add 2 tsp powdered chocolate peanut butter.
- Measure a 0 point amount of peanuts, by weight (2.5 gm), then crush them and set aside. For me, it was 3 peanuts.
- Measure a 0 point amount of chocolate chips, by weight, then place them in a ziplock bag and crush them. Set aside.
- (optional) Order "peanut butter concentrated extract" from Amazon. Replace the 1 tsp of vanilla extract with 1/2 tsp peanut butter extract. It costs a few bucks... but you will deeefinitely be making this multiple times. Or... just use vanilla extract, like normal.
- Right before placing the ramekins into the oven, sprinkle the crushed chocolate and peanuts over the batter, then bake.
- When done baking, melt a scoop of creamy peanut butter in the microwave, in a small dish, 20 seconds at a time.
- When the peanut butter is liquified, scoop out 1/4 tsp and drizzle the liquid PB over the top of the cake. Done.

Salted Caramel Cake:

Recipe Changes:

- Remove the cocoa powder.
- Add 2 tsp powdered peanut butter (trust me).
- Add 1/8 tsp ground cinnamon
- Replace the vanilla extract with caramel extract, found in the baking/spice aisle/or online.
- Sprinkle top of the batter with coarse salt, right before baking.
- (optional) After baking, smear 1/4 tsp Smucker's sugar free caramel sundae syrup on top of the cake, then dust with the powdered sugar. 1/4 tsp doesn't sound like much... but trust me, it spreads great.

Closing Thoughts

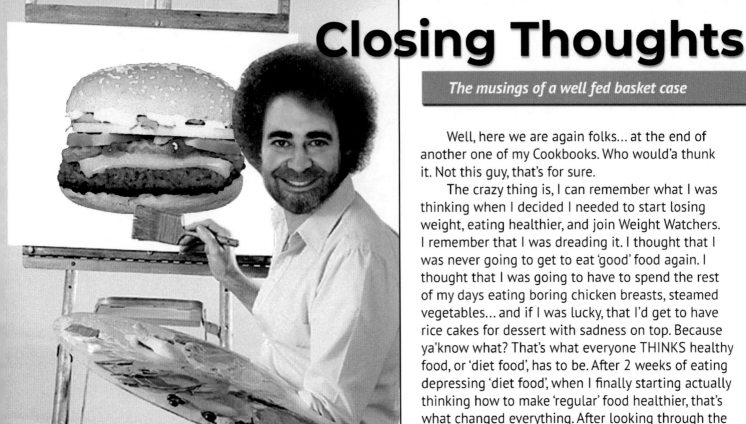

"... and now there's our happy little cheeseburger."

Well, here we are again folks... at the end of another one of my Cookbooks. Who would'a thunk it. Not this guy, that's for sure.

The crazy thing is, I can remember what I was thinking when I decided I needed to start losing weight, eating healthier, and join Weight Watchers. I remember that I was dreading it. I thought that I was never going to get to eat 'good' food again. I thought that I was going to have to spend the rest of my days eating boring chicken breasts, steamed vegetables... and if I was lucky, that I'd get to have rice cakes for dessert with sadness on top. Because ya'know what? That's what everyone THINKS healthy food, or 'diet food', has to be. After 2 weeks of eating depressing 'diet food', when I finally starting actually thinking how to make 'regular' food healthier, that's what changed everything. After looking through the pages of this book, is THIS food that you would have eeeever imagined you could eat and lose weight?

Look at the nutritional info on some of these burgers, a LOT of the fillings on most of these babies have less fat and calories than your typical morning granola bar.... and they're HUGE BURGERS!

In my previous 2 cookbooks, I go out of my way to try and spend time instructing, teaching and guiding you through the steps you can take to modify recipes for yourself. This is my full fledged, straight forward, less jibber jabber Cookbook. I tried to pack as many gourmet burgers and sandwiches into it as possible, as well as give you just shy of 30 dressings and spreads. UTILIZE THOSE DRESSINGS! Don't just think of them as being for these burgers only. Most all of them can be used as salad dressings as well. You can use those to dress potato salads, pasta salads, chopped grilled veggies, etc. Look at the way that I constructed these burgers, then take that process and start creating your own.

Between my 3 self published cookbooks, I've set you up for complete and utter success. You have all of the tutorials, guides and foundation recipes in Cookbook 1. The appetizers, dressings, dips, and all the desserts in Cookbook 2... and now this. Between these 3, there is no way you can NOT lose (or maintain) weight, unless you go completely off the rails and start snacking like a walking vacuum. Don't do it. You don't need to anymore.

At your disposal, you now have: Over 80 sauces, dips, dressings and spreads. A handful of Thanksgiving/Holiday dishes. 20 show stopping appetizers, 37 gourmet and low calorie/fat desserts... and now, 36 restaurant level gourmet burgers & sandwiches. Did I mention the 10 low calorie & fat meat seasoning mixes for ground turkey and chicken? Seriously folks, by this point, you should feel empowered to get cracking in the kitchen, knowing that you are now in charge. You shouldn't ever have to deal with non supportive family members, griping about your 'diet food' ever again. By now, I hope that if I have been able to impart anything after working on these Cookbooks for 2 years, it's that more than anything... I want you to succeed. I don't want to just throw recipes at you. I want to help show you how to create your own. Book 1 explained HOW to do it. Book 2 showed you that you could take it to the next level... and Book 3... this is to show you that just because you might be 'on a diet', doesn't mean you have to eat 'diet food'.

NOW, GET COOKIN'!

Acknowledgements

Well, here we are again. Getting a bit repetitious at this point, but I guess that's a good thing. Seeing that we're at the end of the award show, now's as good a time as any to mention a few key folks. There are a TON of you who have been so extremely supportive and encouraging over the past 6.5 months, while I've been working on this book. Well, if you count the 3 months that we were all shut down because of COVID... I've reeeeeeally only been working on this for 3.5 months, but let's not nit-pick.

Now, let's start with the non-Weight Watchers people. More than any of you realize... a huge reason I was able to put this Cookbook together was because of all the awesome Behavioral Therapists at '**California Psych Care, Santa Clarita**.' These wonderful young women, come to my house, nearly every single day, to help my kids with their therapies. While they are working with my kiddos, that's when I was able to have a small window that allowed me to cook over half of the burgers and sandwiches, as well as set up lights and take pictures. If it wasn't for them, I never would have been able to finish this. I also built over half of the actual book itself during their weekly 'play group' therapy sessions. I'd drop off my kids, sit in their office lobby for 2 hours with my laptop, soak up their wifi and work. Thanks, especially to **Jennifer**, **Stephanie 1**, **Stephanie 2**, **Kendal**, **Olivia**, **Bailey, Melissa** and all the other Therapists and Assistants who have helped my kids be able to communicate ... and have also given me time to cook and work, during the in-home therapies. Thank you, Ladies!

Now... onto the Weight Watchers/Social Media folks. There are a bunch of people, especially in Weight Watchers 'Connect', I want to single out and thank. I won't be able to mention everyone, because there are so many of'ya. But I do have to call out a few. *(C'mon... there's 130,000+ of you following me right now and I only have half a page left!)*.

Of course, I have to start off with **@69gabygal**... the poor lady who has been acting as my Jiminy Cricket for 2 years now. She helps me with proof reading and suggesting changes, nearly every night. Honestly, folks... that lady is thorough. Any mess ups that you find in here, are ones that I've put in AFTER she proof read everything... which I do, a lot. It's a wonder I haven't driven her crazy yet.... Actually, I probably have. Which is why I always tell her I'm going to replace her with a younger Editor, from The Ukraine, named Inga... just to keep her in line. 😂

@Mariarachael12 and her Husband Jodi, for being wonderful to me from the moment I met them. **@Missyvw40**, **@Eastendergirl** and **@AliciawMccauley**. 3 friends that I'm so glad I was able to meet, in person. **@Rbberens**, for being my selfless, local WW friend. **@Bizzybee85, @Cake.Riot, Mecaara**... **@Renelfalgout1**, for being such a great sport and playing along in **#ConnectWars**, as 'The Cajun Queen', along with **@Mappleby777**, for slumming it as the sidekick of my arch nemisis... **@Chiafullo**...'The Cannoli Kid', aka: 'The Lover of Kale.' As well as a somewhat cryptic one...'**Ron**'. Thank you. Thank you for all of the help you have given me and my family over the past 2 years. Thank you, **#GentFromConnect**.

I want to give a special shout out to my absolute 2 favorite little chefs, who I absolutely adore. '**Chef Frankie**', the pint sized cooking dynamo of Connect, son of **@Ericarossiramos**... I still owe you a little chef jacket, haven't forgotten, mi amigo. As well as **@dtspilde**'s youngest daughter, who is cooking her way through all my recipes. *"Go, Team Dull Knife!!!"*

Ya'know what... I'm going to break from tradition here. I want to say thank you to Weight Watchers, for everything. I was going to do it in Cookbook 2, but chickened out. Well, it's about time I said thanks to the corporation that put this system in place. Joining WW changed my life. It changed my family's lives. It gave me the tools and desire to change myself for the better. When I joined Weight Watchers, I was medically classified as Obese. I had a combined cholesterol of over 270, RESTING blood pressure of 180, sleep apnea, pre diabetes, etc., etc., etc. If it wasn't for hitting my 'low' and joining, I would be dead of a heart attack or stroke right now. Instead, because of their system, everything about me changed, not just physically.

For people who haven't really looked into it, Weight Watchers is NOT 'just for grandma'. Look at the 'muy macho' burgers in this book. What red blooded dude wouldn't want to sink his teeth into one of these burgers? Heck, just looking at the nutritional values for this food, by itself, should blow your mind. Look at the type of food that Weight Watchers gives you the tools and ability to create. Want fresh pasta with vodka sauce... and want to lose weight while eating it? That's in Cookbook 1. Want to eat 1/2 cup of Hummus with only 5 grams of fat in it? Cookbook 2. Want a healthier version of a Big mac that only has 6 grams of fat? Page 32. All of this recipe hacking, ingredient swapping, culinary craziness that I do, to make EVERYTHING into healthier 'diet food' ... Weight Watchers didn't show me how to do it. But, they DO provide you with the tools, to figure out HOW you can have almost anything and still lose or maintain weight. So, with that out of the way... Daniel, out. Till next time.

Nutritional Values

One of the biggest reasons for cooking and preparing meals like I do, is because I want to eat amazingly snazzy food, without having to reduce my portions. Most popular food bloggers, "skinny" cookbook authors, and celebrity chefs, usually have tiny, toddler sized portions. That's how they say their food is low calorie. Of course, it is. You're being served a plate fit for Poppa Smurf. In equal amounts, my recipes are usually around 1/2 (or less) of the points, fat and calories of everyone else. Seriously… "Eat a responsible 1/8 cup serving of stuffing…" Umm… that's 2 Tablespoons. No. Wanting to lose weight doesn't mean that you have to eat 'diet' portions.

CONDIMENTS Dressings & Spreads	POINTS 1 serving (G-B-P)	SERVING SIZE	CALORIES	FAT (grams)	CARBS (grams)	SUGAR (grams)	PROTEIN (grams)	PAGE #
5 Minute Marinara	0-0-0	1/4 cup	25	0	5	2	1	14
Asian Chili Aioli	0-0-0	2 Tbsp	15	0	3	2	1	14
Asian Orange Sauce & Glaze	0-0-0	1/2 cup	60	0	14	6	2	14
BBQ Sauce	0-0-0	1/4 cup	20	0	4	2	1	14
Bruschetta	0-0-0	1/4 cup	15	0	3	2	1	15
Buffalo Sauce	0-0-0	1/4 cup	10	0.5	2	0	0	15
Cheese Sauce	4-4-4	2/3 cup	100	15	15	3	9	15
Chick Fil A copycat	1-0-0	1/4 cup	60	1	9	6	2	15
Classic Coleslaw Dressing	2-1-1	2/3 cup	170	4	26	23	8	16
Creamy Italian Dressing	1-0-0	1/4 cup	45	2	5	1	2	16
Creole Remoulade	0-0-0	2 Tbsp	50	3	5	2	1	16
Dark Cherry Sauce	0-0-0	2 Tbsp	60	0	15	5	0	16
Dijon Vinaigrette	0-0-0	1/4 cup	60	1	5	4	3	17
Enchilada Sauce	0-0-0	1/4 cup	15	0	3	1	1	17
Garlic Pepper Aioli	0-0-0	2 Tbsp	35	1	5	3	2	17
Katsu Sauce	0-0-0	1/4 cup	40	0	9	5	1	17
Ketchup	0-0-0	1/4 cup	20	0	4	3	1	18
Lemon White Wine Aioli	1-0-0	1/4 cup	60	1	7	5	3	18
Mango Chili Sauce	0-0-0	1/4 cup	50	0	12	10	1	18
Maple Mustard Spread	0-0-0	2 Tbsp	25	0.5	3	1	1	18
Mayonnaise Substitute	0-0-0	1/4 cup	40	1	5	4	2	19
Mustard Beer Spread	0-0-0	2 Tbsp	25	0	2	1	1	19
Ranch Dressing	1-0-0	1/4 cup	60	1	8	6	4	19
Rice Wine Dressing	0-0-0	1/4 cup	45	1	8	5	2	19
Roasted Garlic Mustard Spread	0-0-0	2 Tbsp	35	0.5	5	3	2	20
Sesame Ginger Dressing	0-0-0	1/4 cup	100	4	13	7	5	20
Smoky Red Onion & Bacon Jam	1-1-1	1/4 cup	50	1.5	7	4	3	20
Teriyaki Sauce	0-0-0	1/4 cup	15	0	3	2	0	21
Thousand Island Dressing	1-0-0	1/4 cup	45	0.5	7	5	3	21

SALADS	POINTS 1 serving (G-B-P)	SERVING SIZE	CALORIES	FAT (grams)	CARBS (grams)	SUGAR (grams)	PROTEIN (grams)	PAGE #
BBQ Ranch Chicken Salad	3-1-1	1 Serving	210	7	15	5	23	108
Blue Cheese Wedge Salad	2-2-2	1 Serving	80	2.5	9	6	5	108
Broccoli Salad	1-1-1	1 Serving	60	1	11	9	3	109
Caesar Salad	5-3-3	1 Serving	140	7	13	5	7	109
Classic Creamy Coleslaw	1-0-0	1 Serving	45	1	7	6	2	110
Cobb Salad	3-1-1	1 Serving	240	10	9	4	26	110
Creamy Garlic & Onion Pasta	4-3-3	1 Serving	160	1.5	34	7	7	111
Crunchy Asian Chicken Salad	2-1-1	1 Serving	150	4	9	5	19	111
Mediterranean Salad (Olive Garden)	1-1-1	1 Serving	120	4.5	16	0	5	112
Mexican 'Street Corn' Salad	6-1-1	1 Serving	190	3.5	37	14	9	112
Mustard & Dill Potato Salad	2-2-0	1 Serving	100	0.5	21	2	4	113

SPECIAL REQUEST:

In early July, the prior versions of my first 2 cookbooks were removed from Amazon. Therefore, I lost ALL of their reviews from the past year and a half. If you could PLEASE leave a review on Amazon for my books, I would greatly appreciate it. Even if you've only ever downloaded them, you can still leave a review on Amazon. The printed books have the same content as the published books. I need all the help I can get to build the ratings back up. Thank you.

SIDE DISHES

SIDE DISHES	POINTS 1 serving (G-B-P)	SERVING SIZE	CALORIES	FAT (grams)	CARBS (grams)	SUGAR (grams)	PROTEIN (grams)	PAGE #
Balsamic Brussel Sprouts	1-1-1	1.5 cups	80	1	17	5	6	100
Creamed Style Sweet Corn	3-0-0	1/2 cup	110	1.5	24	7	3	101
Crispy Baked Onion Rings	1-1-1	1.5 cups	110	3	16	4	5	102
Garlic Dijon Mushrooms	0-0-0	3/4 cup	50	1	7	3	6	103
Loaded Mac n Cheese	3-3-1*	1/2 cup	110	1.5	19	2	6	104
Maple & Bacon Baked Beans	3-1-1	3/4 cup	110	1	20	2	8	105
Parmesan Carrot Fries	0-0-0	1/4 pound	80	1	18	8	2	106
Perfect Potato Wedges	5-5-0	8 large wedges	180	0.5	42	2	4	107

The high amount of carbs in some of my sides and bonus recipes are from my use of erythritol based sweeteners. Other sweeteners have less carbs.

BONUS RECIPES

BONUS RECIPES	POINTS 1 serving (G-B-P)	SERVING SIZE	CALORIES	FAT (grams)	CARBS (grams)	SUGAR (grams)	PROTEIN (grams)	PAGE #
Burger Buns (yeast)	3-3-3	1 bun	100	0.5	21	2.4	2.5	114-115
Cucumber Mint Lemonade	0-0-0	8 oz (1 cup)	10	0	3	1	0	116
Easy Peach Cobbler	3-3-3	2/3 cup	170	1.5	38	6	2	117
Peanut Butter & Jelly Cake	7-6-6	1/12 slice	260	6	46	4	11	118-119
Personal Sized Cocoa Cake	3-3-3	1 mini cake	138	1	65.6*	0.8	4.6	120-121

The 1 gram per serving of sugar in my lemonade recipe is from the natural sugars in lemon juice and cucumber.
36 grams of carbs in my 'cocoa cake' are from my use of erythritol based sweeteners. If you use Splenda or a non erythritol sweetener, the carbs drop dramatically.

BURGERS & SANDWICHES

BURGERS & SANDWICHES	POINTS 1 serving (G-B-P)	SERVING SIZE	CALORIES	FAT (grams)	CARBS (grams)	SUGAR (grams)	PROTEIN (grams)	PAGE #
The All American	3-2-2	1 Burger	150	1.5	20	9	20	24-25
Animal Style Cheeseburger	3-2-2	1 Burger	250	3	32	20	8	26-27
Bacon Mac n Cheese	4-2-2	1 Burger	290	3	28	4	26	28-29
Bahn Mi Burger	5-4-4	1 Burger	160	3.5	24	15	38	30-31
Big Dan (big mac copycat)	5-3-3	1 Burger	450	6	59	13	44	32-33
Blue Cheese & Onion	4-2-2	1 Burger	310	13	17	10	33	34-35
Bruschetta Chicken	4-2-2	1 Sandwich	200	6	5	3	29	36-37
Buffalo Ranch Chicken	5-3-3	1 Sandwich	260	7	15	9	33	38-39
Chicken Club	4-2-2	1 Sandwich	220	7	6	4	31	40-41
Chicken Cordon Bleu	4-3-3	1 Sandwich	340	11	21	8	37	42-43
Chicken Parmesan	4-3-3	1 Sandwich	330	10	17	3	40	44-45
Chick Fil A copycat	3-2-2	1 Sandwich	320	8	20	9	39	46-47
Cod Sandwich 'The Codfather'	2-0-0	1 Sandwich	190	3	16	11	24	48-49
Crispy Fish Sandwich	3-1-1	1 Sandwich	240	5	21	10	27	50-51
Enchilada Burger	1-0-0	1 Burger	130	1.5	15	8	17	52-53
French Bistro	5-3-3	1 Burger	170	6	6	3	22	54-55
Gastro Pub	6-2-2	1 Burger	300	11	11	5	40	56-57
Green Chili Chorizo	1-0-0	1 Burger	120	1	12	5	16	58-59
Havana (Cuban)	3-2-2	1 Burger	210	7	12	5	24	60-61
Jerk Chicken	1-0-0	1 Sandwich	370	6	19	15	60	62-63
Juicy Lucy	3-2-2	1 Burger	180	2	8	3	33	64-65
Kafta (Lebanese)	2-1-1	1 Burger	150	3	15	5	7	66-67
Meatloaf Sandwich	5-3-3	1 Sandwich	380	14	21	11	36	68-69
Mushroom & Swiss	5-3-3	1 Burger	210	2.5	13	7	33	70-71
Oktoberfest (German)	2-1-1	1 Burger	140	4.5	7	2	18	72-73
Orange Chicken	2-1-1	1 Sandwich	290	6	26	10	33	74-75
Patty Melt	5-3-3	1 Burger	160	4	12	6	21	76-77
Pizza Burger	3-2-2	1 Burger	210	8	15	4	20	78-79
Reuben Burger	4-2-2	1 Burger	190	7	4	2	28	80-81
Salmon Burger	5-1-1	1 Burger	280	8	20	10	29	82-83
Sausage & Peppers	2-1-1	1 Burger	200	8	18	6	16	84-85
Shrimp Po'Boy	2-1-1	1 Sandwich	220	4	14	3	32	86-87
Sloppy Joe	2-0-0	1 Sandwich	200	2	15	8	31	88-89
Teriyaki	1-0-0	1 Burger	170	1.5	27	17	15	90-91
Thanksgiving	3-2-2	1 Burger	220	2.5	33	12	20	92-93
Western Bacon Cheeseburger	5-3-3	1 Burger	180	3.5	17	8	22	94-95

Book Index

A Roadmap For The Madness

A
All American Burger ... 24-25
Animal Style Cheeseburger ... 26-27
Asian Chili Aioli ... 14
Asian Orange Sauce & Glaze ... 14

B
Bahn Mi Burger (Vietnamese) ... 28-29
Bacon Mac n Cheese Burger ... 30-31
Balsamic Glazed Brussel Sprouts ... 100
Basic Mac n Cheese ... 30
BBQ Ranch Chicken Salad ... 108
BBQ Sauce ... 14
Big Dan & Junion Dan Burger ... 32-33
Blue Cheese & Onion Burger ... 34-35
Blue Cheese Wedge Salad ... 108
Bonus Recipes:
    Burger Buns ... 114-115
    Cucumber Mint Lemonade ... 116
    Easy Peach Cobbler ... 117
    Peanut Butter & Jelly Cake ... 118-119
    Personal Sized Cocoa Cake ... 120-121
Broccoli Salad ... 109
Bruschetta ... 15
Bruschetta Chicken Sandwich ... 36-37
Buffalo Ranch Chicken Sandwich ... 38-39
Buffalo Sauce ... 15
Burger Buns ... 114-115
Burgers & Sandwiches ... 24-95
Burgers:
    All American ... 24-25
    Animal Style Cheeseburger ... 26-27
    Bahn Mi ... 28-29
    Bacon Mac n Cheese ... 30-31
    Big Dan & Junior Dan ... 32-33
    Blue Cheese & Onion ... 34-35
    Enchilada ... 52-53
    French Bistro ... 55-55
    Gastro Pub ... 56-57
    Green Chili Chorizo ... 58-59
    Havana (Cuban) ... 60-61
    Juicy Lucy ... 64-65
    Kafta (Lebanese) ... 66-67
    Mushroom & Swiss ... 70-71
    Oktoberfest ... 72-73
    Patty Melt ... 76-77
    Pizza ... 78-79
    Reuben ... 80-81
    Salmon ... 82-83
    Sausage & Peppers ... 84-85
    Teriyaki ... 90-91
    Thanksgiving ... 92-93
    Western Bacon Cheeseburger ... 96-97

C
Caesar Salad with Croutons ... 109
Caramelized Onions ... 32
Cheese Sauce ... 15
Chicken Club Sandwich ... 40-41

Chicken Cordon Bleu Sandwich ... 42-43
Chicken Parmesan Sandwich ... 44-45
Chick Fil A copycat ... 15
Chick Fil A Sandwich ... 46-47
Classic Coleslaw Dressing ... 16
Classic Creamy Coleslaw ... 110
Cobb Salad ... 110
Cod Sandwich ... 48-49
Condiments, Dressings & Spreads ... 14-21
    Marinara ... 14
    Asian Chili Aioli ... 14
    Asian Orange Sauce ... 14
    BBQ Sauce ... 14
    Bruschetta ... 15
    Buffalo Sauce ... 15
    Cheese Sauce ... 15
    Chick Fil A Sauce ... 15
    Classic Coleslaw Dressing ... 16
    Creamy Italian Dressing ... 16
    Creole Remoulade ... 16
    Dark Cherry Sauce ... 16
    Dijon Vinaigrette ... 17
    Enchilada Sauce ... 17
    Garlic Pepper Aioli ... 17
    Katsu Sauce ... 17
    Ketchup ... 18
    Lemon White Wine Aioli ... 18
    Mango Chili Sauce ... 18
    Maple Mustard Spread ... 18
    Mayonnaise Substitute ... 19
    Mustard Beer Spread ... 19
    Pico De Gallo ... 52
    Ranch Dressing ... 19
    Rice Wine Dressing ... 19
    Roasted Garlic & Mustard ... 20
    Sesame Ginger Dressing ... 20
    Smokey Red Onion/Bacon Jam ... 20
    Teriyaki Sauce ... 21
    Thousand Island Dressing ... 21
Creamed Style Sweet Corn ... 101
Creamy Italian Dressing ... 16
Creamy Italian Veggie Pasta Salad ... 111
Creole Remoulade ... 16
Crispy Fish Sandwich ... 50-51
Crunchy Asian Chicken Salad ... 111
Cucumber Mint Lemonade ... 116

D
Dark Cherry Sauce ... 16
Dijon Vinaigrette ... 17

E
Enchilada Burger ... 52-53
Enchilada Sauce (red) ... 17

F
French Bistro Burger ... 54-55

G
Garlic Dijon Mushrooms ... 103
Garlic pepper Aioli ... 18
Gastro Pub Burger ... 56-57
Green Chili Chorizo Burger ... 58-59

H
Havana Burger (Cuban) ... 60-61

I
Important Ingredients ... 10-11
Important Kitchen Gadgets ... 9

J
Jerk Chicken Sandwich ... 62-63
Juicy Lucy Burger ... 64-65

K
Kafta Burger (Lebanese) ... 66-67
Katsu Sauce ... 17
Ketchup ... 18

L
Lemon White Wine Aioli ... 18
Loaded Mac n Cheese ... 104

M
Mango Chili Sauce ... 18
Maple & Bacon Baked Beans ... 105
Maple Mustard Spread ... 18
Marinara Sauce ... 14
Mayonnaise Substitute ... 19
Meatloaf Sandwich ... 68-69
Mediterranean Salad (olive garden) ... 112
Mexican 'Street Corn' Salad ... 112
Mushroom & Swiss Burger ... 70-71
Mustard & Dill Potato Salad ... 113
Mustard Beer Spread ... 19

N
Nutritional Information ... 124-125

O
Oktoberfest Burger (German) ... 72-73
Onion Rings ... 102
Orange Chicken Sandwich ... 74-75

P
Parmesan Carrot Fries ... 106
Patty Melt Burger ... 76-77
Peach Cobbler ... 117
Peanut Butter & Jelly Cake ... 118-119
Perfect Potato Wedges ... 107
Personal Sized Cocoa Cake ... 120-121
Pickled Veggies ... 28
Pico De Gallo ... 52
Pizza Burger ... 78-79
Potato Salad ... 113

Q

R
Ranch Dressing ... 19
Reuben Burger ... 80-81
Rice Wine Dressing ... 19
Roasted Garlic Mustard Spread ... 20
Roasted Tomatoes ... 67

S
Salads:
    BBQ Ranch Chicken Salad ... 108
    Blue Cheese Wedge Salad ... 108
    Broccoli Salad ... 109
    Caesar Salad ... 109
    Classic Creamy Coleslaw ... 110
    Cobb Salad ... 110
    Creamy Roasted Garlic & Onion Pasta Salad ... 111
    Crunchy Asian Chicken Salad ... 111
    Mediterranean Salad (olive garden) ... 112
    Mexican 'Street Corn' Salad ... 112
    Mustard & Dill Potato Salad ... 113
Salmon Burger ... 82-83
Sandwiches:
    Bruschetta Chicken ... 36-37
    Buffalo Ranch Chicken ... 38-39
    Chicken Club ... 40-41
    Chicken Cordon Bleu ... 42-43
    Chicken Parmesan ... 44-45
    Chick Fil A ... 46-47
    Cod Sandwich *'The Codfather'* ... 48-49
    Crispy Fish ... 50-51
    Jerk Chicken ... 62-63
    Meatloaf ... 68-69
    Orange Chicken ... 74-75
    Shrimp Po'Boy ... 86-87
    Sloppy Joe ... 88-89
Sausage & Peppers Burger ... 84-85
Sesame Ginger Dressing ... 20
Shrimp Po'Boy ... 86-87
Side Dishes:
    Balsamic Brussel Sprouts ... 100
    Creamed Style Sweet Corn ... 101
    Crispy Baked Onion Rings ... 102
    Garlic Dijon Mushrooms ... 103
    Loaded Mac n Cheese ... 104
    Maple & Bacon Baked Beans ... 105
    Parmesan Carrot Fries ... 106
    Perfect Potato Wedges ... 107
Sloppy Joe Sandwich ... 88-89
Smokey Red Onion Bacon Jam ... 20
Stuffing/Dressing ... 92

T
Teriyaki Burger ... 90-91
Teriyaki Sauce ... 21
Thanksgiving Burger ... 92-93
Thousand Island Dressing ... 21

U

V

W
Western Bacon Cheeseburger ... 94-95

X

Y
You... should write a review ;-)

Z

Daniel Von Lichtinstein, 5th Earl of Hamburg
1690 - 1749 • Creator of the Modern Hamburger
(Photo courtesy of the Lichtinstein Trust)

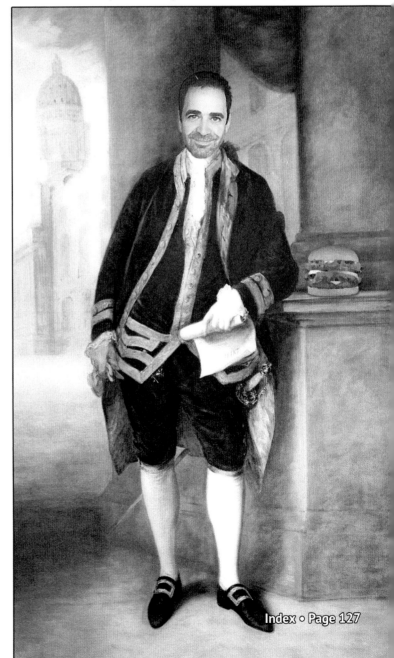

Made in the USA
Columbia, SC
19 October 2020